Jits van Straten

Ashkenazic Jews and the Biblical Israelites

Jits van Straten

Ashkenazic Jews and the Biblical Israelites

The Early Demographic Development of East European Ashkenazis

DE GRUYTER
OLDENBOURG

This book was generously sponsored by
The Eduard van Straten Funds
The Irène Bollag-Herzheimer Stiftung
Marijke Borchardt en Jan Baart
Ineke Pey

ISBN 978-3-11-070128-9
e-ISBN (PDF) 978-3-11-070138-8
e-ISBN (EPUB) 978-3-11-070149-4

Library of Congress Control Number: 2020947875

Bibliographic Information published by the Deutsche Nationalbibliothek
The Deutsche Nationalbibliothek lists this publication in the Deutsche Nationalbibliografie; detailed bibliographic data are available on the Internet at http://dnb.dnb.de.

Cover illustration: The Meneptah stele, an Egyptian inscription which mentions a people named Israel. Wellcome Library, London, CC BY 4
Printing and binding: CPI books GmbH, Leck

MIX
Papier aus verantwortungsvollen Quellen
FSC
www.fsc.org
FSC® C083411

www.degruyter.com

For Sven,
a gifted archaeologist who had to put up with much unwarranted criticism

Acknowledgements

This book would not have come about without the help of others.

I would like to offer special thanks to Martin Richards (University of Huddersfield) for his helpful discussions and critical reading of the chapter on DNA.

The employees of the sector special collections of the library of the University of Amsterdam were exceptionally helpful, thank you very much.

Thanks are due to Sophie Kohler (Ben-Gurion University of the Negev), who not only reviewed the manuscript, but also provided useful material that improved the book.

I also want to extend my thanks to my editor, Julia Brauch, for the pleasant cooperation. John Ryan and Lydia Burns did the copy editing. Thanks very much for all the work.

Last, but not least, I want to thank my friend Dini Venema for all the time she spent on reviewing the manuscript and providing useful comments.

https://doi.org/10.1515/9783110701388-001

Contents

List of Figures and Tables

Figures

Tables

https://doi.org/10.1515/9783110701388-002

Glossary

Ancient DNA (aDNA)	DNA isolated from ancient biological materials
Approximate Bayesian Computation (ABC)	Approximate Bayesian Computation constitutes a class of computational methods rooted in Bayesian statistics
Autosomal DNA	DNA not involved in sex determination, located on the autosomal chromosomes
Founder effect	A reduction in genetic variation that results when a small part of a population starts a new population
Genetic admixture	The presence of DNA in an individual from a distantly-related population as a result of interbreeding
Genetic bottleneck	Sharp reduction in the size of a population due to a disaster or migration, resulting in a sharp reduction in the genetic diversity (comparable to founder effect)
Haplogroup	A group of similar haplotypes that share a common ancestor
Haplotype	A haplotype is a set of DNA variations within a haplo-group that tend to be inherited together
Mitochondrial DNA (mtDNA)	Mitochondrial DNA is the small circular chromosome found inside mitochondria. The mitochondria are organelles found in cells that are the sites of energy production. Mitochondria, and thus mitochondrial DNA, are inherited from mother to offspring
Multidimensional scaling (MDS)	A means of visualizing the level of similarity of individual cases of a dataset. It is the same as principal coordinates analysis
Mutation	A mutation is a permanent heritable change in a DNA sequence
Phenotype	Physical and/or biochemical characteristics of a person
Principal component analysis (PCA)	PCA is a mathematical procedure that transforms a number of (possibly) correlated variables into a (smaller) number of uncorrelated variables called principal components
Single nucleotide polymorphism (SNP)	A DNA sequence variation that involves a change in a single nucleotide

Y Chromosomes

The Y chromosome is one of two sex chromosomes. Humans and other mammals have two sex chromosomes, the X and the Y. Females have two X chromosomes in their cells, while males have X and Y chromosomes in their cells. Egg cells contain an X chromosome, while sperm cells contain an X or a Y chromosome. This arrangement means that during fertilization, it is the male that determines the sex of the offspring

Introduction

The study of the beginnings and origin of specifically East European Ashkenazic Jewry becomes an unrewarding activity when one finds out that the nowadays accepted hypotheses about this origin are not tenable and should be revised. These hypotheses pertain to 1. the beginnings of German Jewry during the ninth to the tenth century; 2. the mass migrations from Germany to Eastern Europe during the Middle Ages; and 3. the resulting explosive population increases of East European Jewry between 1500 and 1800 (explosive, according to European criteria for that period).

With regard to the beginnings of Ashkenazic Jewry, the decree by Emperor Constantine in 321 that the Jews also had to be represented in the city council (*curia*) appears to be generally accepted by Jewish and non-Jewish history scholars. For example, "There is not a shred of doubt that at the beginning of the fourth century, the city of Cologne had a Jewish community, not only that, this community must have been important" (Baltrusch 2002, 4). Following a negative remark about an early Jewish presence in Brittany, Toch (2001, 12) writes (translated from German):

> Likewise, the situation is not much better in the Germanic provinces. At the beginning of the fourth century, as emphasized by a written source, there was an organized and mighty Jewish community in Cologne [...] a second [...] general law by Emperor Constantine in 330 certainly cannot have anything to do with Cologne.

According to the currently accepted hypothesis, a continuous Jewish presence started during the second half of the ninth century (for example, Toch 1994; Toch 1998, 5; Ostrer 2012, 21; Xue et al. 2017). It denies a continuous Jewish presence in Cologne between 321–330 and the ninth century.

What are the arguments? There is no information about a Jewish presence between 321 and the ninth century. I want to emphasize that Jewish history scholars appear to agree on the presence of a well-developed Jewish community in 321, despite the fact that there is no information about this community available from the period before 321. Was the Jewish community flown in maybe by Alitalia on the day of the decree? According to Weinreich (1980, 320–330) the reason for the lack of information between 330 and the ninth century is the violent arrival of the Franks (Germanic tribes) who caused the Jews to flee to Gaul. However, Weinreich's view is subject to scrutiny. First of all, the take-over was not that violent, as can be seen by the lack of burned material in the old city wall. Second, Cologne had a mixed Roman-Germanic population long before the fourth century. Third, why would the Franks who were not yet Christians

https://doi.org/10.1515/9783110701388-003

have more problems with the Jews than with the rest of the population? Fourth, nothing is known about groups who left, so why, all of a sudden, the Jews? All this makes it very unlikely that an important Jewish community disappeared just like that without a clear-cut reason. Not every historian is convinced of the currently accepted hypothesis. Caro (1908, vol. 1, 159) assumes that the Jews may have continued to live in Cologne, similarly to the situation in Gaul, but the confirmed history of German Jewry only started in the tenth century. A similar careful view is expressed by Breuer and Graetz (1996, 19) who are of the opinion that continuity cannot be excluded. A much more logical explanation for the lack of information may well be that in 881 the Vikings invaded Cologne, and destroyed the city archives (Gechter and Schütte 2000, 118). For Toch (1998, 80) the issue of continuation is clear (translated from German): "Modern research has settled the romantic idea of continuous Jewish settlement from the classical antiquity until the Middle Ages [...] the regularly advanced presence of Jews in late Roman Cologne and perhaps also in other places, is irrelevant for the further development." However, German Jewry started much earlier or, put differently, it continued, as was shown by the oldest archaeological information about Cologne reported by Kraus and published by Kober (1945) in the Proceedings of the American Academy for Jewish Research, in which he discusses the archaeological work by Otto Kraus in 1922. According to Kober, Kraus was well acquainted with the field of Roman antiquities. The work was in the form of a manuscript and had not been published. I will follow Kober's discussion of the article rather extensively, as it is relevant for the discussion of an early Jewish presence in Cologne. The site of excavation was the *Judenbüchel,* the "height of the Jews". The *Judenbüchel* in Cologne consisted of an elevation rising a few feet above the land surrounding it. It is identical with the old Jewish cemetery.

In 1922 the mount was used to enlarge the freight yard at the Bonn Gate. During the necessary groundwork, human bones in Roman graves and old stone walls were found. The Jewish community requested to have the bones removed. According to Kraus, the oldest Jewish cemetery in Cologne had been uncovered: "The cemetery tract apparently embraced 29,200 square meters; 6,800 were dug up by the contractors of the railroad; 11,400 were uncovered by the archeological excavations [...] the cemetery had been in use since Roman times". Thus, Kraus did not excavate the whole area. This is noteworthy, as we will see further on. This ancient Jewish cemetery is identical with the medieval Jewish cemetery as far as the location is concerned. It was not a pagan cemetery, nor a Roman-Christian cemetery, and also not a medieval Christian graveyard:

> [...] the orientation of the skeletons in an east-west direction, the position of the hands at the sides and the occurrence of Hebrew tombstones, when considered in connection with the documentary evidence from the twelfth century, left no doubt that this was actually the most ancient Jewish cemetery in Cologne.

Kraus concluded that the graves are from after 270 CE. However, not everybody agreed with Kraus's conclusion, such as Fremersdorf, who became director of the Roman and Germanic Division of the Wallraf-Richartz Museum in 1923. Further on, I will refer to Fremersdorf again with regard to the dating of body graves excavated in 1937. However, after Kraus had checked his material once more, he stuck to his conclusion that the graves belonged to the Roman and subsequent periods up to and including the Middle Ages. When viewed critically, there is no conclusive reason for rejecting Kraus' interpretation. Without going into the whole discussion, Kober concludes that:

> it is possible to assume that the vaulted and stone-covered graves come from the late Roman period or, in view of the fact that the Roman occupation ended about 400, from the fifth or sixth century at the latest [...] Although we cannot determine the exact period from which the stone-covered graves of the Jewish cemetery come, we may at least assume with Otto Kraus that, in general, the Jewish cemetery outside the Bonn Gate dates back to late Roman times.

The discovery by Kraus is also mentioned by Schuler (2004, 469) and Harck (2014, 522–523).

There is more information about the early presence of Jews in Cologne that, to the best of my knowledge, has not been referred to earlier in connection with our subject. Fremersdorf (1938/39) reported the excavation of two body graves from the first to third centuries CE at the corner of the Bonner and Raderberger Strasse in Cologne. The location is part of the Roman graveyard adjacent to the late antique Jewish cemetery. His assertion agrees with his conclusion about the 1922 excavation mentioned above. The question is, how reliable is this conclusion? In the State Archive, file BA R 58/9002, Bl. 336 (see Simon 2006, http://homepages.uni-tuebingen.de/gerd.simon/VorgeschDossiers.pdf) is an evaluation of Fremersdorf by the SD in 1937. The SD was the intelligence agency of the SS and the Nazi party. The evaluation says (translated from German): "Fremersdorf [...] although he is an archaeologist, he is very concerned about emphasising the German elements in the Roman culture in the Rhineland. However, he is ambitious." In view of his positive evaluation by the SD, it becomes questionable how reliable Fremersdorf is when it comes to describing Jewish graves in Cologne. Interestingly, the Fundbücher (documentary files sorted according to the year of excavation) in which the precise data of the excavation are described, present in the Römisch-Germanisches Museum in Cologne, are difficult to be consulted. Schütte (personal communication) writes:

> The archaeologists who were carrying out the work were unaware of the border between the two cemeteries because they had not carried out topographical research beforehand, and the border was not marked. At one point, they dug up two body graves. Unknowingly, they had already entered the old Jewish cemetery. They were graves of persons who had not been cremated, and whose grave had a tent-like tile roof, which is typical for graves of the fourth century (late antique) and especially the Jewish graves excavated by Kraus in the direct vicinity. So, they neutrally described the graves as body graves of the fourth century. In the non-Jewish cemetery, the majority of the graves were cremations or had a different grave architecture. It is, therefore, most likely that they had found Jewish graves. These graves still had bones because Kraus' excavation did not cover this part of the *Judenbüchel* cemetery. We are lucky that the archaeologists did not know that they were Jewish graves because it is inconceivable that they would have reported about a Jewish grave during the Nazi period. So, here we have a clearly documented find of a late antique Jewish grave in Cologne, described in a "neutral" way.

The consequence is that if a Jewish cemetery existed in late Antiquity, what Otto Kraus and Kober already suggested as early as 1922, then the presence of a larger community is obvious. If there would have been a discontinuity in Cologne, the medieval and post-medieval Jewish cemetery could likely not have been in the identical place of the Roman Jewish burial-place. Even more important, a continuity until the late middle ages must then be mandatory (in addition to the evidence resulting from the Carolingian synagogue, as we will see further on). However, modern research presents a contradictory image, namely of discontinuous development.

The late Roman period did not conclude with the end of the occupation in 400 (Dopsch, 1923, vol. 1, 159). It is known that Roman customs were cherished for a long time after 400. The information by Kraus via Kober means that a continuous Jewish presence in Cologne is a serious possibility. As mentioned before, the lack of information about a Jewish presence after 330 does not prove anything, especially when the city archives were destroyed. The finding of the Jewish graves and the lack of a good reason for the departure of only the Jews from Cologne make Toch's denial of a continuous Jewish presence questionable. It also puts Toch's negative remarks about the Constantine decree of 330 in another light, because if it was a general decree it may have applied to Cologne as well. After all, there is no reason to assume that the Jewish community all of a sudden had disappeared in 330.

Until the end of the nineties of the last century, the oldest synagogue of Cologne was thought to have been built at the beginning of the eleventh century. Kober (1934, 71) writes (translated from German): "According to a late tradition, which has little value, the synagogue [...] was built in 1012 or 1040". Kober made a good assessment of the tradition: at the end of the nineties, Schütte (1998, 188–189) published a sensational archaeological discovery: the synagogue was actually a Carolingian synagogue, built on top of an older building, possibly an antique synagogue (Gechter and Schütte 2000, 113). The construction of the synagogue was started close to the end of the eighth century and ended around 881. The city of Cologne must have had a reasonably developed Jewish community at the beginning of the ninth century, otherwise it could not have started to build a synagogue.

At a congress in Frankfurt a/M in 2003, Toch attacked Schütte's archaeological find of a Carolingian synagogue with political arguments. He was obviously unable to refute Schütte's conclusions with archaeological arguments. In addition to the lack of a solid reason for the supposed disappearance of the Jewish community of Cologne during the late Roman period, and the discovery of the late Roman graves by Kraus, the finding of a Carolingian synagogue is another indication of a continuous Jewish presence up to the Carolingian period. It is not clear why Toch is so vehemently against a continuous Jewish presence between the fourth and the ninth century.

With regard to the second hypothesis – East European Ashkenazis originated in Germany – I proposed an alternative origin via southern Ukraine as it is called today. What made me reject the hypothesis that East European Jewry originated in Germany? Briefly, the accepted hypothesis states that during the pogroms of the Middle Ages, between 1096 and roughly 1500, German Jewry migrated to Eastern Europe (Poland and Lithuania). This view is based specifically on the publications by two East European Jewish history scholars, Baron (1957–1976) and Weinryb (1972/1973). I will therefore call it the Baron-Weinryb hypothesis. It is based on assumptions about mass migrations, culminating in the remark by Ankori (1979, 36) that at the end of the Middle Ages "Western Europe was *judenrein* (cleared of Jews)". In order to show how unrealistic Ankori's statement is, I would like to refer to the *Stammbuch der Frankfurter Juden* by Dietz (1907, 343–344), who studied the age of the Jewish and non-Jewish families in Frankfurt a/M, and refers to the situation in his time (translated from German):

> Back to the time of Lüther, only about 20 [Christian] families could be traced back [...] Against this finding, the age of the Jewish community here that I now demonstrated, should be designated as very surprising [...] The following chronological order of Jewish family names shows the solid evidence that among them, not only relatively, but also absolutely, more old families were present than among the remaining population of our city.

He then shows that of the present Jewish families, 33 could trace their roots back to the period between 1316 and 1400, and another 33 to the period between 1400 and 1500.

Despite the fact that there is no evidence for the mass migrations, the Baron-Weinryb hypothesis arrives at the conclusion that East European Jewry originates from Germany. On the other hand, German Jewish history scholars, specifically the authors of the reference work *Germania Judaica*, came to different conclusions about this period. The latter produced a typical German piece of work in the sense that it is *gründlich* (thorough). The number of references to archival sources to back up the content is impressive. However, the work shows no substantial migrations of Jews from Germany (or Bohemia) to Eastern Europe. The conclusion can therefore only be that German Ashkenazis and East European Ashkenazis have a different origin, and thus should not be considered as one population. Despite the lack of evidence for the mass migrations, the Baron-Weinryb hypothesis has become the accepted hypothesis about the origin of East European Ashkenazis. For example, Botticini et al. (2016) do not even mention *Germania Judaica* in their discussion about the origin of East European Ashkenazis.

As a consequence of the abovementioned migrations, the number of Jews in Eastern Europe at the end of the Middle Ages, in 1500, was supposedly rather low because there were not that many Jews in Germany during that period. The arch-fathers of the Jewish population sizes in Eastern Europe in 1500 and 1650 are also Baron and Weinryb. Between 1500 and 1650, the Jewish population increased from 30,000 to 450,000 (Baron 1957, v. 16, 4 and 207) or from 10,000 to 200,000 (Weinryb 1972, 32 and 197). Hundert (1997) sticks to the total of 50,000 Jews in Poland in 1500. It is important to note that there is no factual basis for these population sizes. When we realize that in 1800 there were just over two million Jews in Eastern Europe, the Jewish annual growth rate between 1500 and 1800 must have been explosive, more than one percent (third hypothesis). Relative recently it became clear that according to modern demographers, such population increases were not possible in Europe during that period, which put an end to the third hypothesis as well.

A more recent hypothesis states that East European Jewry originated mostly in the Czech lands, Silesia and the former eastern German provinces (Stampfer 2012, 136–137). I will come back to this hypothesis in chapter 2.

The origin of the Yiddish language is also controversial. The three major hypotheses concerning the origin of Yiddish are the Rhineland hypothesis (Weinreich 1980, 329–330), the Danube hypothesis (Faber and King 1984; Katz 1985), and the Sorb hypothesis (Wexler 1991). In 2011, I suggested that a fourth hypothesis, the Bavarian-Czech hypothesis (Eggers 1998), is more appropriate to explain the origin of Yiddish in Eastern Europe (van Straten 2011a, 115–122).

The consequence of the opposing conclusions of the two approaches to Ashkenazic history, Baron-Weinryb versus *Germania Judaica*, is that I had to decide which historiography to follow. Because the historiography in *Germania Judaica* is superior – it does not include implausible population increases either – I did not have much of a choice. Interestingly, one does not find a thorough discussion in the literature on the differences between the two approaches in historiography. Thus, my rejection of the nowadays accepted Baron-Weinryb hypothesis has nothing to do with a new hypothesis; it is only the result of my decision to consider *Germania Judaica* a more reliable source.

As the Baron-Weinryb hypothesis and the hypothesis by Stampfer about the origin of East European Ashkenazis are still the generally accepted explanations of their origin, most geneticists who study the origin of Ashkenazic Jewry base their research on the abovementioned historians (for example, Behar et al. 2004a; Slatkin 2004; Palamara et al. 2012; Gladstein and Hammer 2019), and thus do not differentiate between German and East European Ashkenazis. This becomes particularly clear when statistic models are used including implausible population increases. Therefore, my choice for *Germania Judaica* also has implications for the evaluation of genetic research pertaining to Ashkenazis: genetic research has to agree now with an origin of East European Ashkenazis that does not imply Germany as the place of origin. In other words, genetic results become questionable if they are based on the "out of Germany" hypothesis with its high population increases.

In view of the discussion so far, I figured that the study of the origin of Ashkenazic Jewry requires a multidisciplinary approach that includes the fields of history, demography, linguistics, archaeology, and genetics. Investigating the combination of these disciplines is not only necessary because all four have something to do with the origin and spread of Ashkenazic Jewry, but also because, as we saw before, studies of each discipline separately led often to controversial results.

I had to try and find another way to explain the origin of East European Ashkenazis. In 2011, I published a partial solution (van Straten 2011a) that showed that, within Europe, East European Jewry migrated from what we call today roughly the region of southern Ukraine into the more northern and western parts of Eastern Europe. A Jewish presence in Eastern Europe around the Black Sea, already before the beginning of the Common Era, is mentioned in the literature. The possibility that these Jews are part of the ancestors of today's East European Ashkenazis is systematically ignored or even denied by almost all historians who deal with this subject. The next questions to be answered were where did these Jews come from, when did they get there, and could they have been ancestors of today's East European Ashkenazis? I tried to provide an answer in an article entitled "The origin of East European Ashkenazim via a southern route" (van Straten 2017). The main conclusion of the article is that the ancestors of East European Jews first came from Anatolia and Greece, and later on from Italy.

However, more questions remained. For example, how do today's Ashkenazis relate to the biblical Israelites genetically? What do the different lineages of today's lay-Jews, Jewish priests, and Levites mean? In order to get answers to these and other questions, I included in this study also archaeological data from the biblical period between about 1200 BCE and the beginning of the Common Era. I decided to follow mainly the archaeological work of Israel Finkelstein, an Israeli top archaeologist, because his realistic conclusions made sense to me. The field of genetics will receive extra attention. This book will be based to some extent on the abovementioned article.

Which authors do I refer to? I do not pretend to have read every article and every book that relates to the subjects that are discussed. To the best of my knowledge, the most important literature is being referred to. Sadly enough, it is not always immediately clear whether or not the information a historian dishes up is true. Wrong information may be the result of an unfounded idea, a misquote, or falsification. This is especially a problem when the information is taken from earlier works. In such a case, one has to check the earlier source. In addition to having come across this phenomenon doing a peer review, I also encountered such a situation when I wrote this book. It was a very frustrating experience, because the information seemed very important. At the end of 2019, I started to read the book *ha-ashkenazim ha-rishonim* (האשכנזים הראשונים –the first Ashkenazis) by Asher Frishman. In the introduction, he writes (translated from Hebrew): "However, people from the east of all people, and especially the heads of the Talmud schools (Hebrew *geonim*, singular *gaon*), already define "*ashkenaz*" as Germany and they mention "Ashkenazis" as Jews who lived in communities in Western Europe." So far, nothing wrong. But then comes the surprise: the information comes from a source written in the ninth century, *seder amram gaon* (the prayer book of Amram Gaon) by Amram ben Sheshna (died ca. 875). This is exciting news, because it shows that in the ninth century there were Jewish communities in Germany (he speaks of Ashkenazis). It seemed too good to be true. I went to the Rosenthaliana, the Judaica library of the University of Amsterdam, and read the book. No *ashkenaz*, no Germany, and no Ashkenazis. I felt, as the saying in German goes, *himmelhoch jauchzend, zu Tode betrübt*. These days, this kind of information would be called fake news. The author was unable to tell me why the book was referred to. I only refer to this book as an example of wrong information, and would not have bothered otherwise. I tried to discuss authors that are representative of the different opinions on each subject. The number of authors discussed varies with the subject. For example, few authors who still follow the Baron-Weinryb hypothesis will be referred to, because enough has been written about this hypothesis. I will quote authors who do not agree with me and also not with the Baron-Weinryb hypothesis.

In chapter I, I will use archaeological data to give a short historical overview of the ethnic composition in Palestine before the beginning of the Common Era, which is a new, necessary topic with respect to the origin of Ashkenazic Jewry. It will be followed by the switch from Judeans (or Israelites) to Jews, and the change in the definition of Ashkenazis from Ashkenazis by descent to Ashkenazis by rites. In chapter II, historical and demographic problems with an origin from Germany, the Czech lands, and the eastern German lands will be discussed. Only the "problematic" topics of the disciplines that were used earlier will be referred to. As to historiography, the controversial results are mainly related to the interpretation of migrations of Ashkenazic Jewry during the Middle Ages. The discussion of demographic aspects will be limited to the outdated data of East European Jewish population increases. Because the field of genetics has become a particularly important field today, chapter III will be dedicated to a discussion of the genetic results that are linked to the Baron-Weinryb hypothesis in one way or another. The chapter will show that it is necessary to combine genetics with reliable historiography and demography. The importance of the German-Jewish literature will conclude the chapter. Chapter IV will deal with historical and genetic evidence for a Jewish presence around the Black Sea before and after the beginning of the Common Era. The question of why East European Jews speak Yiddish will be answered in chapter V. The answer to this question will be narrowed to the phenomenon that a Slavic-speaking Jewish population switched to Yiddish. To show that historical and genetic problems do not occur in Ashkenazis only, the proposition that Turkish Jews are Sephardic Jews (Hebrew: *sefaradim*) will be discussed in chapter VI. The chapter will be followed by a general summary of the forgoing chapters.

Finally, in the epilogue I will give my personal view on what is happening to the discussion about the origin of Ashkenazic Jewry and related subjects.

I Israelites, Judeans, Jews, and Ashkenazis

Israelites

What information do we have about the history and ethnic composition of the early Israelites, or “Emergent Israel” as Leuchter (2017, 36) calls them? Thanks to extensive archaeological research, reliable information about the inhabitants of what was called “Canaan” has become available. Information about this period is necessary in order to understand the genetic relationship between Ashkenazis and these inhabitants, their supposed ancestors.

The first time the name “Israel” appears in an extra-biblical source is on the Merneptah stele from 1207 BCE (see cover). The stele commemorates the victory of pharaoh Merneptah over three cities in Canaan: Ashkelon, Gezer, Yeno‘am, and Israel. The first two are in the coastal region. According to Na‘aman (1977), Yeno‘am was most likely located in Transjordan. He provides three data to make his point plausible. One of them is the Amarna letter *EA* 197. In this letter, Yeno‘am is located in the Bashan region which is in Transjordan. The name “Israel” does not appear as a name of a town or a region. On the stele, it says: “Israel is laid waste, his seed is naught”. Leuchter (2017, 37) concludes from the wording that “it is Israel’s “seed” (i.e., families) [that] has been annihilated”. This oldest source does not give any information about the ethnic composition of “Israel”. Furthermore, it is also not clear what the geographic connection is between “Israel” and the region of the Israelite monarchy that came about at the end of the eleventh century BCE (Finkelstein 1996).

Finkelstein and Silberman (2002, 110–118) showed that the early Israelites started out as nomads, appeared around 1200 BCE as herders in the hills of Canaan, and with time became farmers. Their culture was a simple one of subsistence and was clearly different from that of the lowland Canaanites. Their villages were not fortified, which shows that they had friendly relations with their non-Israelite neighbors. The initial population must have consisted of some 45,000 people, divided over 250 villages. The authors conclude:

> the emergence of early Israel was an outcome of the collapse of the Canaanite culture, not its cause. And most of the Israelites did not come from outside Canaan–they emerged from within it. There was no mass Exodus from Egypt. There was no violent conquest of Canaan. Most of the people who formed early Israel were local people–the same people whom we see in the highlands throughout the Bronze and Iron Ages. The early Israelites were–irony of ironies–themselves originally Canaanites.

https://doi.org/10.1515/9783110701388-004

But, highland Canaanites also have to originate from somewhere, and probably from somewhere different to the lowland Canaanites, because, as mentioned before, their material culture was different.

The origin of the early Israelites is not known. There are no local written sources from that period. There is written information about Canaan in the Amarna letters from the fourteenth century BCE. In these letters, the diplomatic correspondence between the Egyptian and Canaanite authorities, two unruly groups are mentioned, Shosu and Apiru. The Shosu were pastoral nomads, whom the Egyptians called plunderers. During the late fourteenth century BCE, they formed a large portion of the population that lived in the central part of the territory that later would be designated as the kingdom of Judah, especially in the steppe and the highlands. It is not clear what the relationship is between the Shosu and the Israelites. In the Egyptian sources, the Apiru are described as a bunch of outlaws or as mercenaries. Therefore, the name does not refer to an ethnic group. They were the ones who made most of the problems. Finkelstein and Silberman (2006, 42) describe them as

> uprooted peasants and herders who sometimes turned bandits, sometimes sold themselves as mercenaries [...] and were in both cases a disruptive element [...] by either local rulers or the Egyptian administration to maintain the stability of their rule.

The authors wonder whether David, before he became king, could be considered an Apiru chieftain with his gang. This idea is based on the fact that an Apiru chieftain had previously become a political leader and on the resemblance between the biblical stories and the description of the Apiru in the Amarna letters. In their conclusion, they stop short of calling David and his men Apiru. Instead, they write: "The most plausible historical scenario [...] is that an Apiru-like leader known as David emerged as a local strongman at a time of political chaos."

It is clear though, that the early Israelites lived in Canaan for about 200 years before King Saul (1025–1005; Finkelstein and Silberman 2002, 131) appeared on the scene. From a historical point, the only information about the origin of the Israelites comes from the Hebrew Bible: Israelites are descendants of arch-father Abraham. Is the arch-father theory tenable? As an answer to the question at this point, I would like to quote part of the last paragraph of the chapter on the Patriarchs (ibid., 47) in which the authors refer to the Jerusalem version of the *torah:*

> The great genius of the seventh-century creators of the national epic was the way in which they wove the earliest stories together without stripping them of their humanity or individual distinctiveness. Abraham, Isaac, and Jacob remain at the same time vivid spiritual portraits and the metaphorical ancestors of the people of Israel. And the twelve sons of Jacob were brought into the tradition as junior members of more complete genealogy.

Thus, the arch-father idea is not right, but what is the status of the twelve tribes? Are they a metaphor for the ethnic heterogeneity of the different tribes? If the latter is the case, it may show up in genetic research.

We will jump almost one hundred years to an important point in Israelite history, the splitting up of King Solomon's kingdom. In the year 931 BCE, Jeroboam I, son of Nebat, became king of the northern part of the country, while Rehoboam, followed up his father as king of Judah. During this period, the religious practices in the kingdom of Judah were similar to those in the northern kingdom. In Judah

> religious ideas were diverse and dispersed [...] there was the royal cult in the Jerusalem Temple, there were the countless fertility and ancestor cults in the countryside, and there was the widespread mixing of the worship of YHWH with that of other gods (ibid., 246–247).

Due to all kinds of environmental and economic factors the northern state became much more powerful and numerous than the southern state. Between 884 and 842 BCE, the kingdom of northern Israel was ruled by kings of the Omride dynasty: Omri, Ahab, Ahaziah, and Joram. Their territory consisted of Samaria, the mountainous Galilee, Hazor in the upper Jordan Valley, large parts of Transjordan between the Arnon and Yarmuk rivers, and the coastal plain of the Sharon (Finkelstein 2013, 79; see Figure 1):

> The highlands of Samaria–the core territory of the state and the seat of the capital– were inhabited by village communities that would have identified themselves culturally and religiously as Israelites. In the northern lowlands–the Jezreel and the Jordan valleys–the rural population was comprised mainly of settled peasant villages that had been for centuries closely linked to the Canaanite city-states. Farther north were villages more closely aligned to the Aramean culture of Syria and to the Phoenicians of the coast. (Finkelstein and Silberman 2002, 191–92).

Around the middle of the ninth century BCE, King Hazael of Aram-Damascus occupied part of the northern kingdom that the king "claimed were originally Aramean". The authors add that "the population in this part of the Israelite kingdom was partly, if not mostly Aramean". The occupation did not last much longer than a few decennia. After that, Hazael was attacked by the Assyrian king Adad-nirari, who became king in 811 BCE. As a result, Hazael had to give up the occupation of the northern kingdom, which became a vassal state of Assyria though. The kingdom became prosperous around 800 BCE. During the reign of King Jeroboam II (788–747), the size of the total population of the kingdom

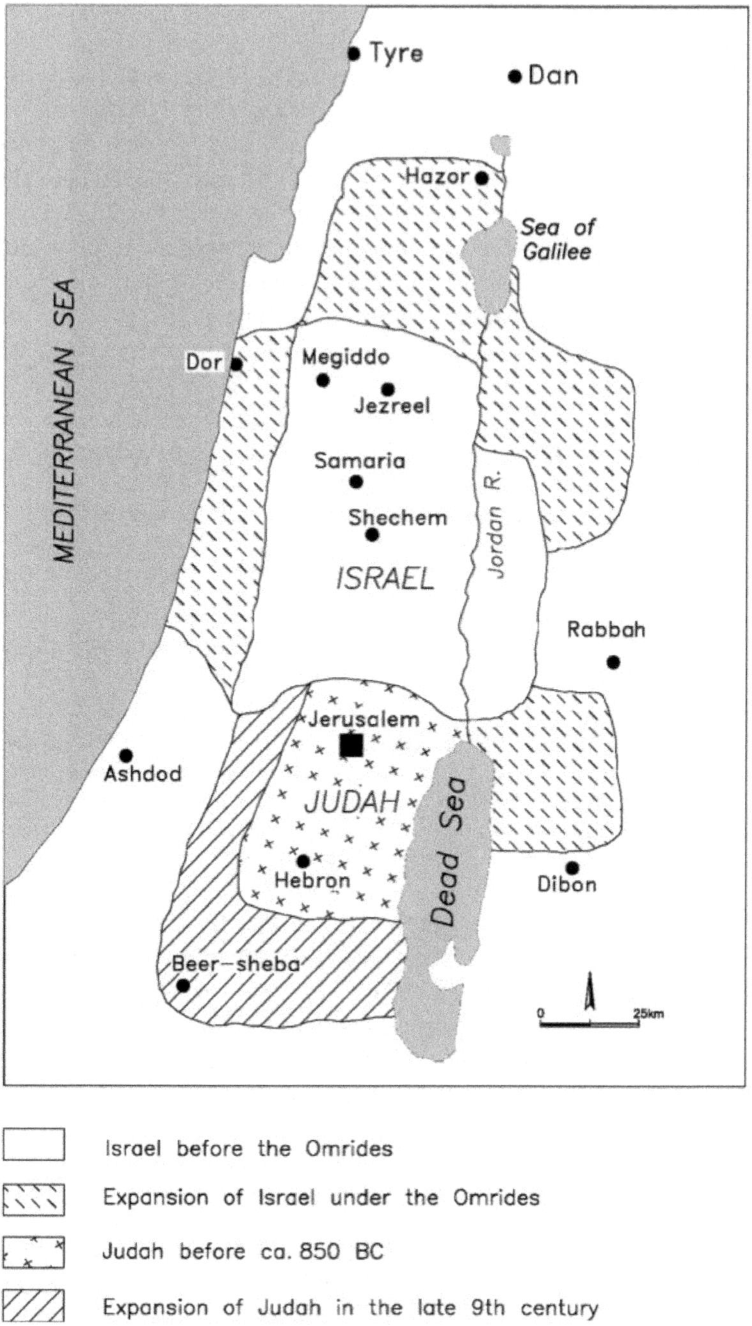

Figure 1: The northern kingdom before and during the Omride dynasty (from Finkelstein 2013, 79).

was about 350,000, while the size of the population of Judah was hardly bigger than 100,000.

In 745 Tiglat-pileser III became king of Assyria. He began to annex the countries between Assyria and the Mediterranean Sea, including the northern kingdom. Because King Pekah (735 – 732 BCE) of the northern kingdom had ended his vassaldom to Assyria, the Assyrian king decided to occupy the northern kingdom as well (ibid., 214–216). Tiglat-pileser III deported part of the population to Assyria and replaced them with new populations from Assyria. "[...] the systematic resettling of new populations in [...] recently conquered territory was intended to expand the overall agricultural output of the empire."

According to the king's annals, 13,500 inhabitants of the northern kingdom were deported to Assyria.

In the annals of King Sargon II (722 – 705 BCE) of Assyria about the deportees from Samaria it says the following (Finkelstein and Silberman 2002, 220):

> I counted as spoil 27,280 people, together with their chariots [...] I formed a unit with 200 of their chariots for my royal force. I settled the rest in the midst of Assyria. I repopulated Samaria more than before. I brought into it people from countries conquered by my hands.

The authors (ibid., 220 – 221) suggest from historical and archeological data that the new settlers

> from rebellious areas in southern Mesopotamia, were settled not only in Samaria but also in the particularly strategic area around Bethel [...] on the northern border of the still-independent kingdom of Judah [...] In addition, a few seventh century cuneiform texts bearing Babylonian names that have been found in Gezer [...] provide tangible evidence of the presence of these deportees in the southwestern territory of vanquished Israel.

In the northern part of the kingdom, the Assyrians left the rural population intact so that they could continue to produce olive oil. This rural population consisted mainly of Canaanites, Phoenicians, and Arameans. But Israelites kept on living in the region of Samaria and Bethel as well. Despite the fact that the rural population was left intact, the deportation is often said to have taken place of the whole population, leading to the "ten lost tribes". Finkelstein and Silberman (2006, 128) write:

> In the eighth century BCE, the population of the northern kingdom living west of the Jordan can be estimated at about 225,000. Even if we were to take Sargon's figure of 27,290 Israelite exiles at face value and add to it the 13,500 Israelites claimed by Tiglath-pileser III to have been deported from the Galilee, the overwhelming majority of the rural Israelite population was not deported.

The story of the ten lost tribes is thus strongly exaggerated.

As a result of the fall of the northern kingdom in 720 BCE, large groups of its inhabitants fled to the kingdom of Judah, and its population "at least doubled, if not tripled". It is not possible to know who these refugees were. Sergi (2017, 381–382) says: "[...] the kingdom of Israel encompassed vast territories [...] These regions inhabited divergent groups [...] "Israelites" were, therefore, only one component of the inhabitants living in the kingdom of Israel [...]." Probably, also prophets and priests from the north took refuge with the kingdom of Judah.

Different deities were not only worshipped in the northern kingdom. In Judah, high places were used to worship various gods:

> [...] priests in the countryside also regularly burned incense on the high places to the sun, the moon, and the stars [...] The condemnations of various Judahite prophets make it abundantly clear that YHWH was worshipped in Jerusalem *together* with other deities, such as Baal, Asherah, the hosts of heaven, and even the national deities of the neighboring lands (Finkelstein and Silberman 2002, 242).

Meanwhile, in the kingdom of Judah, King Hezekiah (727–698 BCE) decided to do away with all the idolatry in the high places, and make the worship of YHWH the only legitimate form, and only in the Temple of Jerusalem (ibid., 250). After the death of the king, the religious situation in the countryside returned to the way it was before Hezekiah's reforms, and also there, Baal, Asherah, and the host of heaven could be worshipped again.

In addition to the non-Israelite people and refugees from the northern kingdom mentioned above, the demographic situation in Judah became more complex when, during the reign of King Josiah (639–609), the Assyrians resettled non-Israelite peoples from towns along the Euphrates in the area of Bethel. One of the problems the king faced was that "of intermarriage with foreign women, which must have been a common practice among the Israelites who survived in the territories of the northern kingdom, among whom the Assyrians had settled foreign deportees" (ibid., 95–96). Intermarriage with non-Israelite women had been a problem all along. In Deuteronomy 7: 1 and 4, seven tribes are mentioned with whom Israelites are not allowed to marry: Hittites, Girgashites, Amorites, Canaanites, Perizzites, Hivites, Jebusites. Most of these tribes probably lived in the area of the once two kingdoms as well. In Joshua 23: 13, the Israelites are warned against marrying the foreign tribes among whom they are living. The warning is repeated in Judges 2: 3. The real reason for the warnings may become clear in 1 Kings 11: 1 and 4, where King Solomon (970–931 BCE) is reported to have all kinds of foreign women (mostly from autochthonous tribes), and to have started to worship other gods because of these women. A similar combination of foreign women and idolatry is found in Malachi 2:

10–12 (end of fifth century BCE?). I would not be surprised if Liverani (2005, 352) provides the actual reason the priests and prophets forbade marrying women of autochthonous tribes: "Well aware of the dominant influence of mothers in the upbringing of children, the priests feared that the spread of mixed marriages would inevitably compromise the stability of the Yahwistic faith and cult." A somewhat related event as far as intermarriage is concerned, although much later, is the forced conversion of the Edomites by Johanan the Maccabean in 125 BCE. The extent of force used is disputed.

In 587 BCE, the Babylonian king Nebuchadnezzar destroyed Jerusalem, which marked the end of the kingdom of Judah. Finkelstein and Silberman (2006, 294) estimate that between 5 and 20 percent of the population was exiled to Babylon, mainly the aristocracy. Again, the rural population was left intact. During the reign of Cyrus II (559–530), the Babylonians were replaced by the Persians, and what was left of the kingdom of Judah became the Persian province of Yehud. The king permitted the exiles from the Babylonian period to return to Jerusalem and rebuild the temple. This information is based on two edicts in Ezra, 1: 2–4 and 6: 3–5. According to Liverani (2005, 252–253) this information is fake:

> These edicts were written and used, in much later times, in order to give prestige and imperial privileges to the temple already built in Jerusalem, and as an answer to the claims of the rival temple in Samaria. [...] The return, in fact, did not take place at the time of Cyrus [...] By 520, [...] an important return took place under the leadership of Zerubbabel [...].

It is not clear how many returned. An interesting number mentioned in the book Ezra (around the fifth century BCE), is the more than 100 foreign wives and their children who came along with their returning husbands. They had to be sent back to their own country! I wonder if this inhuman decree by the prophet was really carried out.

The region north of Yehud became the province of Samaria. "Its mixed population of former Israelites who did not go into exile and of foreign groups resettled in the area by the Assyrians were now known as Samaritans" (Ibid., 226). The inhabitants of Yehud are called *yehudim* in Hebrew, which in English is Jews. However, I will not call the inhabitants "Jews" because, as we will see further on, they are defined differently from the people we call "Jews" today.

The short historical review above shows that the area of both kingdoms was inhabited by a heterogeneous population. Furthermore, the worship of various gods, also by Israelites, should have made intermarriages with the local non-Israelites quite easy. A number of these cases pertaining to non-Israelite women appear in the Hebrew Bible, but they normally refer to women of known male personalities. For example, Zippora, wife of Moses, daughter of the Midianite priest Jethro, Ruth, the Moabite woman who was the grandmother of King David, and King Ahab of the northern kingdom (873–852) who married a Phoenician princess (1 Kings 16:31). With the presence of the different non-Israelite tribes in the country, intermarriage with common people must have occurred as well, but that information is lost. It is also not clear if there was such information at all, because marriage was a private matter. This means that there was not a situation like today, where one has to go to an official institution like a rabbi in order to get married. Neither was there a marriage certificate as we know it since the rabbis instituted such a document. The man paid some form of wealth to the family of the bride, and that was it. Whether or not a prophet liked the choice of the woman was not relevant, if a prophet would know about the marriage at all. The repeated warnings in the Hebrew Bible against intermarriage indicate that this was not something out of the ordinary.

It should be clear that it is very difficult to define the predecessors of the Judeans who lived around the beginning of the Common Era. If they were themselves Canaanites as Finkelstein and Silberman call them, we should make a distinction between them – hill Canaanites – and the lowland Canaanites who were different culturally. First of all, the hill Canaanites may be descendants of Apiru and/or Shosu who were not ethnic entities themselves. Then we have the different non-Israelite tribes that may have added to the composition of the Israelite/Judean population via intermarriages, such as the abovementioned Midianites and Moabites, or the seven tribes the Hebrew Bible mentions with whom Israelites were not allowed to marry, but obviously did. Furthermore, two Assyrian kings resettled people from Assyria in the area of the northern kingdom and the kingdom of Judah (eighth and seventh centuries BCE). These settlers and the Edomites should also be added to the list of possible marriage partners. The only conclusion that can be drawn with certainty is that the inhabitants of the two kingdoms with the Jewish religion were not descendants of arch-father Abraham or any arch-father during the last 3,000 years. Any other conclusion is a question of crystal-gazing.

Judeans and Jews

It is common practice to use the word "Jew" for today's Jews and also for those who lived in the area of both kingdoms before the beginning of the Common Era. When referring to the inhabitants of both kingdoms before 587 BCE, I will use the term "Israelites". Between 587 and the beginning of the Common Era, I will use the term "Judeans", supposedly the ancestors of today's Jews. However, the word

"Judean" should not be interpreted as an inhabitant of the territory of the kingdom of Judah only, but also for an inhabitant of the territory of the northern kingdom before and after its destruction in 720 BCE (Fig. 2). The difference between Judeans and Jews is not well discussed in articles and in most books dealing with Jewish history or Jewish genetics. I will therefore first discuss what the terms "Judeans" and "Jews" imply because of their social and genetic implications.

Judeans formed a patrilineal society, and someone with a Judean father was a Judean (Cohen 1999, 266). The ethnic background of the woman was not important, she became a member of the man's clan.

> Marriage was the non-sacramental, private acquisition of a woman by a man, and the state had little legal standing in the matter. The foreign woman who married an Israelite husband was supposed to leave her gods in her father's house, but even if she did not, it never occurred to anyone to argue that her children were not Israelites. (ibid., 265).

Being a Judean can be compared to someone having a certain nationality determined by his or her father. As mentioned above, in the Hebrew Bible, a number of foreign women are mentioned. I will come back to the phenomenon of intermarriage in the third chapter.

Around the second century CE, the rabbis decided to switch to "Jews" (ibid., 263). A Jew is someone whose mother is of the Jewish faith, leading to a matrilineal society. However, this is not the complete definition. A person who converted to Judaism was and still is considered a Jew as well. In most cases, the reason for conversion was probably intermarriage (genetic admixture – henceforth referred to as admixture), and not the religion as such. Thus, the rabbis introduced a cultural-religious community whose members did not necessarily have to originate from Canaan. They abandoned a system based on men and region and replaced it by a system based on women plus a non-measurable inflow of converts. It is not known why the rabbis switched to "Jews". Cohen (ibid., 285–307) discusses the various reasons that have been proposed quite extensively, but he cannot provide a definite reason either. As mentioned on p. 16, the reason may have to do with the upbringing of the young children by the woman. The rabbinical ruling is applied in today's Israel as well. An interesting implication of the rabbinical ruling is that for the rabbis, religion is actually the only decisive factor. A Judean (or Israelite) origin plays no role anymore.

It is not clear to what extent the rabbinical ruling prevented Jews who had remained in their homeland from marrying "non-Jewish" women. However, what happened when Judeans or Jews went to live abroad? There are no numerical data about people who converted to Judaism. The more than 100 foreign

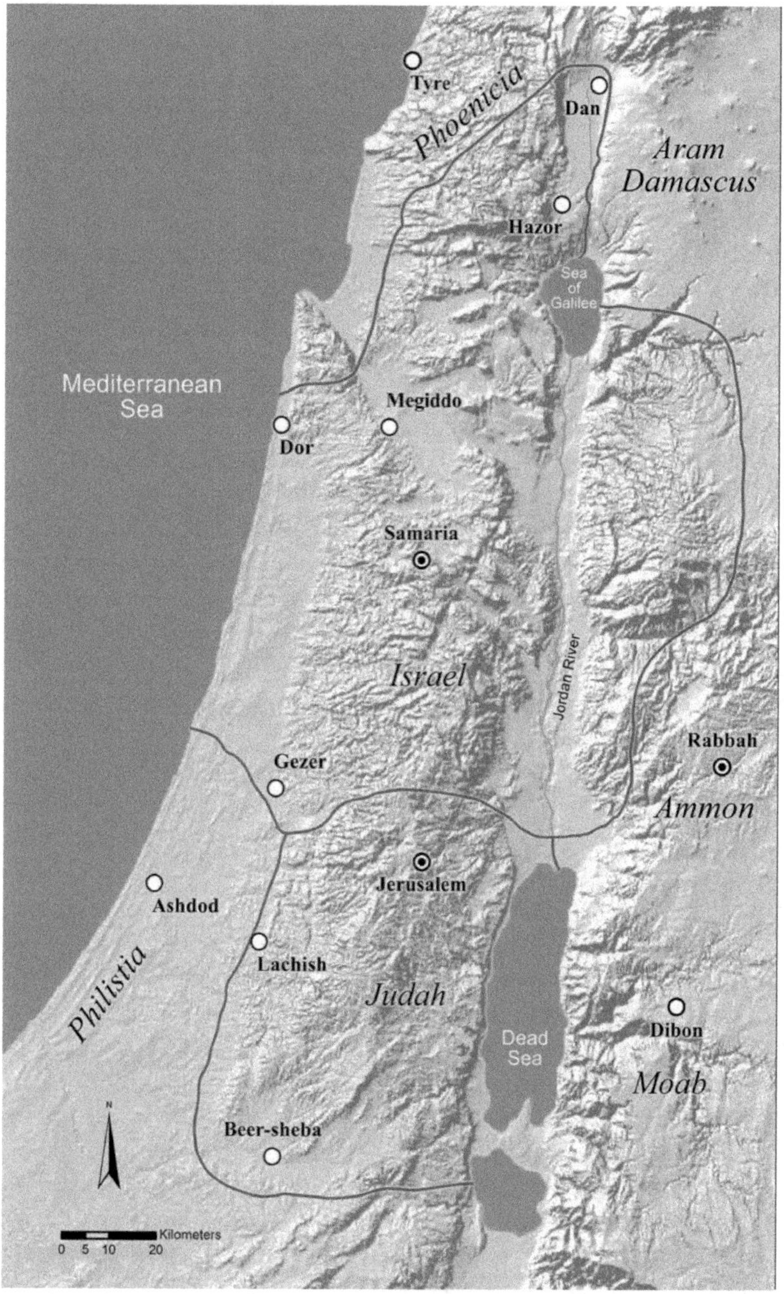

Figure 2: Map of Israel and Judah in the eighth century BCE (from Finkelstein 2013, 2)

women (and children) mentioned above are no proof of conversion either. They are only proof of admixture. Why should these women have converted to the religion of their husbands if this was not an issue in those days? Only after the rabbinical ruling, the conversion becomes a prerequisite for marriage with a non-Jew(ess). Because Judeans started to migrate to other countries well before the rabbinical ruling, there may not have been any official conversion at all. In addition, the conversion took place mainly in the case of marriage after the rabbinical ruling had been implemented, and in such cases, there was no need to register such marriages, because they were simply part of the ruling. It is thus virtually impossible to obtain numerical information about the extent of conversion. We can get a much clearer idea about conversion/admixture by looking at the physical appearances (phenotypes) of today's Jews in different regions. For example, Indian, Chinese, Ethiopian, and European Jews resemble non-Jewish Indians, Chinese, Ethiopians, and Europeans, respectively. The only conclusion that can be drawn is that admixture (conversion) must have been quite extensive. Interestingly, I did not find Jewish history scholars who point toward the obvious connection between admixture and phenotype. When humans migrated to other places their progeny does not adopt the physical features of the autochthonous population without massive admixture. Despite the phenotypic resemblances, Jewish geneticists do not consider European Jews as Europeans. On the other hand, colored Indian and Ethiopian Jews are considered descendants of converts (Behar et al. 2008)!

Thus, in order to differentiate between the differently defined Judeans and Jews, I use the term "Judeans" for the period between 587 BCE and the beginning of the Common Era. The term also agrees with the word the Greeks used, for example, συναγωγὴ τῶν Ἰουδαιῶν (the community of the Judeans). The same holds true for the Roman literature, for example, *Iudaeorum seditio* (the uprising of the Judeans). The use of "Judeans" or "Jews" in this book has nothing to do with the cultural aspects involved. It only pertains to the composition of the group. The Romans considered Judeans and Jews as a cultural group because of their religion but used the geographical name for both of them. A similar use of words is found in the Netherlands where Dutch-born children of Moroccan immigrants are still called Moroccans by many people. The precise date of the switch from Judeans to Jews is not important. If the rabbinical ruling would have been accepted later, for example in some remote areas, it would only have been easier for Judean/Jewish men in these areas to marry foreign women, as had been the custom for centuries. They would still be seen as belonging to a cultural group. The reason for the two terms is only the genetic aspects of the rabbinical switch, leading from a geographically defined group to an ill-defined group.

Ashkenazis

German Jews had specific rites (Hebrew: *nusah ashkenaz*). These rites became the "official" rites of European Jewry, excluding of course the Iberian (Sephardic) Jews. As a result, Jews outside Germany who followed Ashkenazic rites are called Ashkenazis as well. Thus, there are two kinds of Ashkenazis: Ashkenazis by descent, those whose ancestors originated from Germany, and Ashkenazis by rites, those whose ancestors came from somewhere else, for example from Anatolia or Italy, bypassing Germany (van Straten 2017).

Jewish geneticists follow East European Jewish history scholars and treat Ashkenazis as a homogenous genetic population. This is not so strange, because most Ashkenazis live in the United States and Israel, and are for the most part of East European origin. This has led to remarks about Ashkenazic genetic diseases, which are essentially East European Jewish diseases, for example Tay-Sachs disease (Risch 2001). As I mentioned in an earlier publication (van Straten 2011a, 174–177), the TSD carrier frequency among Dutch Jews and probably also German Jews is not higher than that among non-Jewish Dutch or Germans. A relatively recent example of a publication that pooled Ashkenazic Jewry is the article by Guha et al. (2012) about health and diseases among Ashkenazis. (see p. 55).

In chapter 6, I will show that rabbis and possibly teachers of religion were responsible for taking the Ashkenazic rites to Eastern Europe. It is not likely that the few common Jews who migrated from Western Europe eastward were able to make East European Jewry follow Ashkenazic rites. They were no authority, and they also lacked the knowledge to pass on all the laws pertaining to religious life.

Conclusions

1. Early Israelites appeared around 1200 BCE as nomads in the hills of Canaan, and are possibly descendants of Shosu and Apiru, two ethnically undefined groups.
2. The population of Canaan between 1200 BCE and the beginning of the Common Era was ethnically heterogeneous.
3. The northern kingdom of Israel consisted of Israelites and non-Israelite tribes that were indigenous to Canaan.
4. The northern kingdom was much bigger, more populous, and much more powerful than the kingdom of Judah, especially during the dynasty of the Omrides.

5. The story of the ten lost tribes is grossly exaggerated; between roughly 70 to 90 percent of the population remained.
6. Because of the widespread idolatry, intermarriage with non-Israelite tribes occurred.
7. In addition to members of the seven tribes Israelites were not allowed to marry, but probably did, intermarriage could also have taken place with Phoenicians, Medianites, Moabites, and Edomites.
8. The rabbinical ruling that replaced Judeans (based on the "nationality" of the father) by Jews (based on the religion of the mother plus converts), became an additional reason for the inflow of "foreign" people, especially in the diaspora, shown clearly by the geographically determined appearances of Jews in different parts of the world.
9. The rabbinical ruling, in combination with the heterogeneity of the people of Judea, is a disaster for a geneticist who tries to link modern Jews to a fixed group, Judean or other, before the beginning of the Common Era.
10. There are two groups of Ashkenazis: descendants of German Jewry and descendants of Jews who follow Ashkenazic rites.

II History and Demography of East European Jews According to the Baron-Weinryb Hypothesis

Introduction

As mentioned before, the nowadays accepted hypothesis regarding the origin of East European Jewry is the Baron-Weinryb hypothesis. Followers of this hypothesis, with small deviations, are historians like Ben-Sasson, Toch, Hundert, Stampfer, and Bartal, who determine the state of affairs regarding the origin of Ashkenazic history. I will discuss the historical and demographic problems that are attached to this hypothesis. The second view, an origin from Khazaria, will be discussed briefly. For more information, see van Straten 2011a, 5–21.

Germany

The second dubious point I mentioned in the introduction of the book was the substantial Jewish migration from Germany to Eastern Europe (for more information see King 1992; van Straten 2004). The third one was the unlikely high growth rate, 1 percent or more, of the Jewish population in Eastern Europe between 1500 and 1800. At the time Baron and Weinryb wrote their books on Jewish history they could not know that their assumptions as to the fast increases of the East European Jewish population after 1500 would not agree with the opinion of modern experts in demography. Their population increases between 1500 and 1650 lead to exponential growth rates of 1.7 to 2.0 percent. The small population sizes and their growth rates have become a dogma in East European Jewish history. These population sizes are defended by Jewish history scholars and geneticists despite the fact that according to experts in the field of demography there were no population increases of 1 percent or more in Europe for extended periods before 1800. DellaPergola's East European Jewish population sizes lead to exponential growth rates of more than 1 percent as well between 1500 and 1800 (DellaPergola 2001, 22). As these growth rates have become a hot issue, they warrant a more extensive discussion.

A first question that might arise is if the Jewish growth rates are not plausible, how come almost no historian criticized them? There are three answers:

a. Baron and Weinryb showed the Jewish population increase only. If they had shown the growth rate of the total population between 1500 and 1650, 0.22

https://doi.org/10.1515/9783110701388-005

percent, the reader probably would have become suspicious because the Jewish population lived under the same environmental conditions as the non-Jewish population. Figure 3 shows how unlikely Jewish increases are. It is noteworthy that it does not make a difference where in Europe one is; the slow growth rates are virtually the same everywhere.

b. These growth rates were not published in any of the authoritative demographic journals.

c. As said before, these population sizes and growth rates have become more or less a dogma.

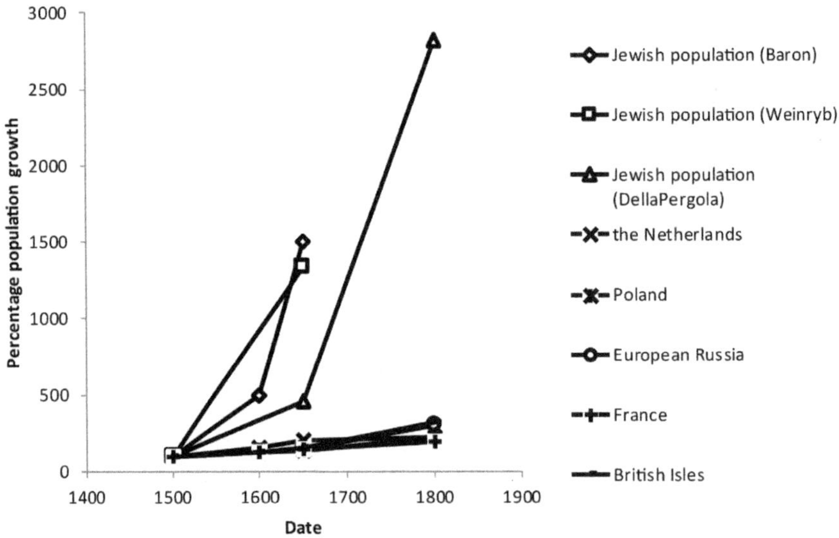

Figure 3: Jewish population growth in the Polish-Lithuanian Commonwealth, 1500 – 1650, according to Baron (1957 – 1976b) and Weinryb (1972, 32), and 1500 – 1800, according to DellaPergola (2001, 22); population growth of the Netherlands, Poland, European Russia, France, and the British Isles, 1500 – 1800 (1500=100 percent; van Straten 2017).

The situation becomes even more incomprehensible when one realizes that there are no reliable numerical data about the size of the Jewish population in Eastern Europe before the census of 1897. Russian non-Jewish history scholars like Binstock and Novoselsky (1915) and Kabuzan (1992) who dealt with Jewish population increases do not have numerical evidence for their high Jewish growth rates either. As they do not add anything to the discussion, they will not be discussed here.

Most arguments used to defend the high growth rates between 1500 and 1800 were refuted in an earlier publication (van Straten 2007). One of the arguments, the use of model life tables, should be explained more extensively. DellaPergola (2001, 22) defends the exceptionally high growth rates by referring to the West model life tables of Coale and Demeny (1966) because "they better fit populations with relatively low child mortality." The West models "were based on mortality experience recorded in populations known to have relatively good vital statistics [...] the tables underlying the 'West model' are a residual collection after the 'East', 'South', and 'North' tables have been removed" (Coale and Demeny 1966, 14). Half the number of life tables underlying the West model are from the twentieth century (52 percent). The remaining ones are taken from the period between 1870 at the earliest and 1960 at the latest. The environmental conditions, in the broadest sense of the word, before 1800 were so much worse than those in the twentieth and late nineteenth centuries that one cannot use the model for the determination of growth rates between 1500 and 1800. In addition, the registration of vital data in Russia was so unreliable that there are no underlying life tables from Russia in the East model. Finally, there are no reliable vital statistics of the Jewish community in Eastern Europe, including child mortality before 1800. Thus, a model is chosen according to some preconceived idea that lacks the necessary vital statistics, and that results in implausible growth rates of one per cent or more. Amazingly, growth rates that are two to four times as high as those of the total population are accepted by Jewish history scholars without question.

Still today, most Jewish linguists and geneticists accept the ideas of Baron, Weinryb, and DellaPergola without verifying or discussing the validity of these increases with experts in demography. Most of the linguists dealing with Yiddish do not bother at all with Jewish population increases – R.D. King (1992) of the University of Texas at Austin is a favorable exception – and the geneticists simply accept them.

There is one more argument used to make the high growth rates plausible that should be mentioned. Stampfer (2012, 136) defends a Jewish annual growth rate of 1.7 percent in Eastern Europe between 1500 and 1700 via a comparison with the high growth rates of the ancestors of the French Canadians: "These numbers [on which the growth rates are based] do not *prove* that the Jewish population grew at a similar rate. They show only that such growth is possible". Obviously, such growth is possible, but not under completely different, worse environmental conditions (the same holds for the Afrikaners he mentions). Anthony Wrigley of Cambridge University, in response to a question about a growth rate of more than 1 percent before 1800 (personal communication), says:

> It was very rare to reach such a rate in pre-industrial times. There are a few exceptions. Rates of growth in colonial North America were such as to double the population in about 30 years, a combination of high fertility brought about by early marriage and low mortality with the bulk of the population widely scattered at low densities, and with unlimited new land to be taken up. But back in Europe rates of increase of 1% p.a. were rare and not long sustained. If the Jewish population which you have in mind was largely urban such a rate is even less plausible. Most towns and cities were dependent on substantial in-migration flows even to maintain their numbers.

The Jewish population in Eastern Europe was indeed mainly urban. The problem with historians who allow for these kinds of high growth rates is that they do not seem to realize that there is a strong relationship between environmental conditions and growth rate.

A second phenomenon that must be mentioned with regards to Jewish population increases is the so-called Jewish demographic miracle of the nineteenth century. This miracle refers to the fact that in both Eastern and Western Europe, the Jewish population increased twice as fast as the non-Jewish population (Ben-Sasson 1976, 790). The miracle and the data of the earlier Ashkenazic population increases have one significant point in common: in neither case is the growth rate of the non-Jewish population shown in the literature. But the miracle has the advantage that it can be checked (van Straten and Snel 2006). There was no such miracle. In regions with reliable Jewish population sizes, the Jewish population increased somewhat faster than the non-Jewish population, but not twice as fast (see also Silbergleit 1930 and Toury 1977, 9–27).

For a more realistic quantitative development of East European Jewry, see Table 1. In this table, the development of East European Jewry is proposed in relation to the development of the total population. The population size of each population in 1800 was the starting point for the calculations leading to the table because the population size in this year was the earliest Jewish population size that could be calculated using relatively reliable Jewish population sizes during the nineteenth century. For the population increases of the Jewish population, two growth rates were used: one according to that of the total population, and one faster, based on the somewhat faster growth of the Jewish population during the nineteenth century. All Jewish population sizes were obtained by calculating back, as shown by two examples (c and d).

Table 1: The total and Jewish population in Russia and Poland: 1–1800.[a]

Total population			Jewish population		
Year	Number	% growth	Number[b]	Number (fast growth)	% (of the total population)
1800	48,193,000			2,050,000	4.3
		0.6			
1700	26,000,000		1,108,100	919,300[c]	3.5
		0.3			
1600	20,000,000		852,400	705,800	3.5
		0.2			
1500	16,000,000		681,900	467,400	2.9
		0.2			
1000	5,200,000		221,400	56,300[d]	1.1
		0.08			
1	2,450,000		105,400	3,700	0.2

a. Total population according to Maddison (2002, 232), Jewish population according to my own calculation (van Straten 2017).
b. Same percentage growth as the total population.
c. Growth of Jewish population$_{1700-1800}$ /1.0062^{100} (growth of total pop.$_{1700-1800}$) = 1.013^{100} (growth of Jewish pop.$_{1800-1900}$)/1.013^{100} (growth of total pop.$_{1800-1900}$) = 2.2. Between 1700 and 1800, the Jewish population increased 2.2 times.
d. Growth of Jewish pop.$_{1000-1500}$/1.0023^{500} (growth of total pop.$_{1000-1500}$) = 1.013^{500} (growth of Jewish pop.)/1.011^{500} (growth of total pop.) = 8.3. Between 1000 and 1500, the Jewish population increased 8.3 times.

The population sizes of the Jewish population in different years differ slightly from those in an earlier table (van Straten 2011a, 98) because in the earlier table I deviated from Maddison's data (which I shouldn't have). It is interesting to note that in 1930, Arthur Rupin (1876–1943), a German-Jewish scientist, calculated the number of Ashkenazis in different periods, and he found an annual growth rate of 0.4 percent between 1500 and 1800. This is actually the same as I calculated for the same period, with the same growth as that of the total population in Russia and Poland. A plausible population increase, certainly for that period.

The consequence of calculating back is that at any time a number is calculated, it may include people of different origins. For example, for the year 1000 the calculation includes not only the number of Jews whose ancestors lived in the region around the Black Sea at the beginning of the Common Era, but also Jews whose ancestors arrived from other places such as Byzantium. It should therefore be clear that the number of Jews calculated for the beginning of the Common Era is too high if it pertains to the region around the Black Sea. Unfortunately, it is not possible to know how many Jews came from Anatolia or Byzantium because numbers are not mentioned anywhere. For the numerical development of East European Jewry, it is not really important.

Czech Lands and the Former German Eastern Territories

In the introduction of the book, we saw that according to Stampfer, East European Jewry mainly originated in the Czech lands, Silesia, and the former German eastern territories, during the period after 1550:

> [...] about three thousand Jews lived in the Czech lands in the mid-sixteenth century [...] these numbers mark the upper limit as to how many migrants could have come from this particular country. The Jewish population of Prague and in the Czech lands grew in the sixteenth and seventeenth centuries. Therefore, only a small minority of the population could have migrated to the east [...] this would have been enough.

Does this hypothesis make migration from western or central Europe more acceptable?

According to Livi-Bacci (1999, 191), estimates of population sizes in 1500 may be off by 20 percent. Assuming that this also holds for 1550, the number of East European Jews would be 574,360 ± 114,870. This would leave us with 459,500 or 689,300 East European Jews in 1550, assuming fast growth. All the 459,500 ancestors and their descendants are needed to end up with the 2 million Jews in Eastern Europe in 1800.

As to Silesia and the German eastern territories, Silesia is part of these territories. There are two options for the location of these territories: they are part of Eastern Europe, or they are not part of Eastern Europe. In the former case, we are dealing with a migration within Eastern Europe. In the second case, one has to know the size of the migration to Eastern Europe. In either case, Stampfer's reference for the migration from these territories, the doctoral thesis of Bürstenbinder (2010, 233–250), is of no help because he does not provide information about the number of Jews in these territories, where they came from, or where they went to.

Let us assume, for the sake of argument, that all of these 459,500 ancestors would have moved to Eastern Europe in 1550. It does not make a difference as to the exponential growth rate whether they all go at once, or via a continuous slow migration, as long as all the descendants contribute to the 2 million. In 1550, the size of the Jewish population in Germany was somewhere between 51,200 and 86,000 with fast and slow growth, respectively (van Straten 2007). To the best of my knowledge, there are no reliable data about the size of the Jewish population in the former German territories or about their migrations. The maximum number of German Jews that could have migrated is 86,000 – 51,200 = 34,800. This would leave enough Jews in Germany to maintain a realistic growth rate of the German Jews. In addition, 3,000 Jews came from the Czech lands, and 421,700 or 651,500 must have come from the former German territories only if they are considered as not being part of Eastern Europe. These numbers cannot be taken seriously, and they become even larger when fewer Jews migrated from Germany. If only a small number of all these Jews would have migrated as Stampfer proposes, we would again end up with implausible exponential growth rates. His proposal does not make a migration from western or central Europe more acceptable.

Finally, Stampfer mentions that the basis for a Silesian origin are German surnames indicating a city, "that are rare enough to be noteworthy". However, such a name does not necessarily mean that the bearer of the surname originated from that city. The name may be used because the bearer of the name had commercial or other ties with that city (Dietz 1907, 8; Bahlow 1953, 78). Under the Habsburg Emperor Joseph II (1740 – 1790), "Jews were ordered to adopt personal and family names (July 23, 1787) (for the most part German ones [...]" (Silber 2017, 791 – 792). To be certain that the Silesian Jews indeed came from Silesia, one should carry out genealogical research about the name bearer. To the best of my knowledge, this was not done.

Rome

According to Zoossmann-Diskin (2010), East European Ashkenazis started their European migrations in Rome, because of the genetic relationship with today's Italians, and because conversions to Judaism were common in ancient Rome. Recently, it was shown that according to mitochondrial DNA (mtDNA) both West and East European Ashkenazis started in Southern Europe, and that there was a genetic difference between West and East European Ashkenazis (Costa et al. 2013). I will come back to Southern Europe as a possible origin in chapter 5.

Given the small number of Ashkenazis in other parts of Western (or Central) Europe during the Middle Ages, East European Ashkenazis cannot have originated there either. This assessment reinforces the existence of Ashkenazis by descent and Ashkenazis by rites. Other possible regions from where some East European Ashkenazis may have originated in Europe are Byzantium and the region around the Black Sea. The former is referred to by some historians, for example, Starr (1939) and Altbauer and Taube (1992). A Jewish presence in the region around the Black Sea dates back to before the beginning of the Common Era. The possibility that East European Jews are to some extent descendants of these Jews is not mentioned in the modern literature. I will come back to this in chapter 4.

Khazaria

The view that East European Jews are partly or mainly descendants of Khazars was proposed by several of authors (for example, Kutschera 1910; Polak 1941; Koestler 1976; Sand 2009). Recently, geneticist Elhaik (2012) also favored a Khazar ancestry. The subject is controversial, and most Jewish history scholars (Landau 1944; Ankori 1979, 19–22; Toch (1998, 80); Stampfer (2013) reject the idea because they argue that an origin not from Judea will have political implications. For example, Stampfer (ibid.) writes: "This carries political implications with regard to the ties between contemporary Jews and the Land of Israel." I will come back to this issue in the epilogue. I will discuss only the article by Elhaik, because he is the first geneticist to compare the Khazar hypothesis with the Rhineland hypothesis, based on DNA research, and the article received a lot of media attention. I must remark though, that the Khazar issue has received more attention than it deserves, as we will see next. Elhaik's conclusions are as follows:

> Our findings support the Khazarian Hypothesis depicting a large Caucasus ancestry along with Southern European, Middle Eastern, and Eastern European ancestries, in agreement with recent studies and oral and written traditions. We conclude that the genome of European Jews is a tapestry of ancient populations including Judaized Khazars, Greco-Romans Jews, Mesopotamian Jews, and Judeans and that their population structure was formed in the Caucasus and the banks of the Volga with roots stretching to Canaan and the banks of the Jordan.

The article rejects a mainly Middle Eastern Jewish origin and thereby deviates from the conclusions by most geneticists.

Before discussing the historical/demographic assumptions on which Elhaik based his conclusions, I would like to mention three methodological problems with the article.

1. A major problem is the very low number of Jewish subjects, for example, one French, three Dutch, and three Austrian Jews.
2. The classification of the Dutch Jews is equivocal. First, they are included with Central European Jews, while in the admixture analysis they are grouped with East European Jews.
3. The three Austrian Jews are themselves a demographic problem.

It is known that before Galicia was annexed by Austria in 1772, the Jewish population in Austria proper amounted to about 8,000 people only (Karniel 1986, 104). The Jewish population of Bohemia, Moravia, and Hungary, which then also belonged to Austria, together amounted to 150,000. In 1772 another 200,000 to 250,000 Jews entered the area of Hungary, Bohemia, Moravia, and Austria. Russian Jews ended up in Austria via Hungary, Bohemia, and Moravia as well (ibid., 105). Of whom are the three Austrian Jews descendants? Without genealogical research, it is not known if we are dealing with Austrian Jews or with originally East European Jews. Statistically, the latter is more likely.

Discussion of Elhaik's Assumptions

"The Khazar Empire existed already in the late Iron Age in the central-northern Caucasus". The first time the Khazars appear in the literature, is in ca. 670 CE when they moved south into the region of the Samara river, about 1,000 km north of the Caucasus. The aforementioned date is far past the late Iron Age (ca. 650 BCE), which means that it is unlikely that the Khazars had an empire in the Caucasus in the late Iron Age.

"The Khazars converted to Judaism in the 8th century". King Bulan of the Khazars converted to Judaism in the ninth century, in 861 (Zuckerman 1995). It is unknown how many Khazars joined in the conversion. Therefore, even apart from the wrong period, there is no evidence for Elhaik's assumption that the Khazars converted in any century.

"Caucasus Georgians and Armenians are considered as proto-Khazars". Considering Georgians and Armenians as proto-Khazars is not based on genetic research, is not so formulated by the authors referred to by Elhaik, and is not in agreement with reliable information about the Khazars. Genome-wide data from non-Jews living in the regions where the Khazars presumably lived showed no evidence for a Khazar ancestry of East European Jews. Kopelman et al. (2009) keep their options open because they detected some similarities in the Adygei. However, it is unknown if the ancestors of today's Adygei had any contact with Khazars. In addition, according to Behar et al. (2013), genome-wide data showed no evidence of a Khazar origin for Ashkenazis. Costa et al. (2013) showed that the major K lineages found among Ashkenazic Jewry do not occur in the Caucasus (including Adygea, located in the Caucasus), and the same holds for the minor Ashkenazic lineages. They concluded that "There is no evidence in the mtDNA pool to support the contention that lineages might have been recruited on a large scale from the North Caucasus [...] as would be predicted by the Khazar hypothesis".

"Prior to their exodus, the Judeo-Khazar population was estimated to be half a million in size". An estimate of half a million Jewish Khazars, or any estimate for that matter, has no factual basis.

"Because, according to both [the Khazar and Rhineland hypotheses], Eastern European Jews arrived in Eastern Europe roughly at the same time (13th and 15th centuries)". The thirteenth-century appears to refer to the collapse of the Khazar Empire. Elhaik seems to be unaware of the Jewish presence in the region of the Black Sea already from before the beginning of the Common Era. There are no sources that show that these Jews disappeared during the first millennium CE. The fifteenth century refers to the expulsions of Jews from the bigger cities in Germany, which according to Elhaik amounted to 50,000 Jews. As mentioned earlier, the expulsions did not lead to migrations to Eastern Europe. Moreover, the number of 50,000 has no factual basis and would have left virtually no Jews in Germany, while the expulsions continued during the sixteenth century.

"Following the collapse of their Empire [...] the Judeo-Khazars fled eastwards [...], settling in the rising Polish Kingdom and Hungary [...] and eventually spreading to Central and Western Europe". Going east one arrives in Kazakhstan and Mongolia. Except for a few Jewish refugees from Khazaria in Toledo around the eleventh century, nothing is known about Jews migrating from Khazaria to Western Europe. Moreover, Jews from Khazaria do not necessarily have to be converted Khazars.

The historical and demographic inaccuracies by Elhaik, together with the conclusions by Behar et al. and Costa et al. refute an important genetic link between (East) European Jews and Khazars.

In the next chapter, I will show that the historical and demographic problems mentioned above caused problematic conclusions in genetic research pertaining to Ashkenazic Jewry as well. This is why the controversial conclusions from genetics will be discussed in the next chapter.

Conclusions

1. There is no historical evidence for mass or gradual migrations from Germany and/or Bohemia before 1500, migrations that could not have been large enough to cause plausible population increases anyway.
2. It is not possible to use the West model life tables of Coale and Demeny to justify population increases of more than 1 percent of East European Jewry before 1800.

3. Demographic data of the ancestors of French Canadians cannot be used to justify the high population increases of East European Jewry before 1800 because the environmental conditions differed too much.
4. A Khazar origin cannot be proven and is also unlikely because Jews lived in the region around Crimea more than 600 years before the Khazars appeared, and more than 800 years before King Bulan converted to Judaism.

III Controversial Conclusions from Genetics

Introduction

The historical and demographic problems mentioned in the previous chapter have their repercussions on genetic research pertaining to Ashkenazic Jewry. This is to a large extent due to the fact that Jewish researchers, who are mostly East European by origin, follow the flawed historical assumption that East European Jewry originates from Germany and Bohemia, a scenario that involves implausible population increases. It is also possible that they are not familiar with modern demography. Furthermore, an important reason for controversial results pertaining to all Jewish groups may well be the lack of historical knowledge of the period before the beginning of the Common Era.

A cause for controversial conclusions of a completely different order is the involvement of politics. The avenue that is followed nowadays in genetics is well worded by geneticist Ostrer (2012, 220):

> The stakes in genetic analysis are high. It is more than an issue of who belongs in the family and can partake in Jewish life and Israeli citizenship. It touches on the heart of Zionist claims for a Jewish homeland in Israel. One can imagine future disputes about exactly how large the shared Middle Eastern ancestry of Jewish groups has to be to justify Zionist claims.

Such a statement is obviously against scientific ethics because it asks for manipulation. Science cannot be mixed with politics. I will come back to this subject in the epilogue.

As long as genetic research has been carried out pertaining to the origin of today's Jews, the results have been controversial and disputed. This holds true for research with mitochondrial DNA (mtDNA) (Thomas et al. 2002; Behar et al. 2006; Costa et al. 2013), Y-chromosomal DNA (Skorecki et al. 1997; Zoossmann-Diskin 1997; Hammer et al. 2000; Zoossmann-Diskin 2000, Behar et al. 2017), and autosomal DNA (Zoossmann-Diskin et al. 2002; Kopelman et al. 2009; Need et al. 2009; Atzmon et al. 2010; Behar et al. 2010; Xue et al. 2017; Gladstein and Hammer 2019).

Genetics of Ashkenazis is inextricably bound up with their history (migrations) and demography. Contradictions may, therefore, have their origin not only in the interpretation of genetic data but also in the interpretation of historical and demographic data. The latter become important when genetic research is combined with these two disciplines, which is normally the case.

Via a number of articles pertaining to mitochondrial, Y-chromosomal, and autosomal DNA, I will show that the controversial status of Jewish genetics is

https://doi.org/10.1515/9783110701388-006

due to several different factors: the importance of the biblical history as the basis for Jewish history before the beginning of the Common Era, the acceptance of converts as part of the religious definition of Jews, and the combination of genetics with disputable historical and demographic assumptions. I would like to end this chapter with a phenomenon that is connected with genetics, but is not being investigated: the blond European Jews.

Historical and archaeological data pertaining to the period BCE showed that the biblical story about the arch-fathers is not tenable and that the priests are not descendants of one forefather. In this chapter, we will find out if genetic research follows archeology or the biblical story. Because Jews are defined via the mother, I will start with three articles pertaining to mtDNA.

Studies with Mitochondrial DNA (mtDNA)

Mitochondria are the small organelles that provide us with energy. Originally, mitochondria were bacteria that entered the eukaryotic world. They are effectively haploid and may have more than one DNA copy (*haplós* is single in Greek; the bacterial genome consists of a single molecule). Mitochondrial DNA is normally inherited from the mother. This means that we can follow the maternal line. The mtDNA that I inherited from my mother ends with me. My children, boys, have the mtDNA of their mother but are also unable to pass it on. Because mtDNA undergoes mutations, and mtDNA with the latest mutation also carries the earlier mutations, geneticists have been able to make a family tree of mtDNA. The tree goes back to the theoretical Eve, and does not consist of names but combinations of letters and numbers, and is divided into groups (lineages or haplogroups) depending on the mutations. To make the information not too technical, I will use mainly "lineages". Each group starts with a letter. For our discussion, the K lineage is the most important. When different mutations take place in women carrying the K lineage, the mtDNAs of the descendants having these different mutations are named lineages K1, K2, K3, etc. When mutations appear among their descendants once more, their mtDNA's are named K1a, K1b, or K2a, K2b, etc. With more mutations in further generations, the naming system continues in such a way that alternately numbers and lowercase letters are alternately used, for example, K1a1b1, which is a major lineage of K1a.

Number of Founding Mothers and their Origin

Thomas et al. (2002) reported that only a few women were involved as founding mothers of 9 geographically separated Jewish groups. However, there is no indication that these founding mothers showed notable genetic similarity.

Behar et al. (2006) suggested that the four major mtDNA founder lineages of today's Ashkenazis, K1a1b1a, K1a9, K2a2a, and N1b, can be traced back to four founding mothers who probably originated in the Middle East. These lineages hardly occurred among non-Jewish populations.

A fundamentally different result was obtained by Costa et al. (2013) who showed that K1a1b1a, K1a9, K2a2a, and N1b are actually European lineages and that this conclusion also holds for most of the minor lineages. The data in Table 2 show that just over 80 percent of the maternal lineages of Ashkenazic women have a European origin (41 + 40.7 percent).

Table 2: Percentages of European and other maternal lineages among Ashkenazis. Major and minor lineages are only provided for the European lineages (based on Costa et al. 2013, Figure 10).

			Lineages			
European				Middle Eastern	Asian	Unassigned
Major	%	Minor	%	%	%	%
K	31.8	H	20.5			
N1b	9.2	J	6.3			
		HVO	4.1			
		T	3.0			
		U	2.2			
		W	1.6			
		I	1.3			
		M1	0.7			
Total	41		40.7	8.3	1.1	9.9

Only 8.3 percent is of Middle Eastern origin, while 1.1 percent is of Asian origin, and 10 percent is not assigned to any region. As to lineage H, Yacobi and Bedford (2016) showed that 3 lineages within the European lineage H7 are found among Ashkenazic Jews. Due to intermarriage with the heterogeneous population in the territory of the two kingdoms, it is not possible to conclude to what group the Middle Eastern mtDNAs belonged.

What is the reason for the difference between the results of Thomas and Behar, compared to those of Costa? Thomas et al. and Behar et al. looked only at the mutations mentioned, while Costa et al. employed a genealogical approach by looking at the "parent" lineages as well. The finding by Costa et al., that the ancestral K1a1b1 is a European lineage, has been confirmed several times for different regions of Europe. Haak et al. (2015) showed that K1a1b1 was found in ancient DNA of a Middle Neolithic individual (3900 – 3600 BCE) in Spain (Supplementary Information section 2, Table S2.1). Knipper et al. (2017) reported the remains of a Bronze Age human skeleton at Wehringen-Hochfeld, Germany with K1a1b1 g (SI Appendix Fig. S3). Olalde et al. (2019) also found human remains with K1a1b1 in Iberia (Supplementary Materials, Table S1), for example, in Alcoi, Alicante (3960 – 3710 BCE), in Granada, Andalucía (2200 – 2000 BCE), and in Valladolid, Castilla y León (1368 – 1211 BCE). Interesting in this respect is the lack of K1a1b1 in non-European Jews and Samaritans (inhabitants of the northern kingdom). This could mean that the Samaritans are maybe descendants of the Israelites. Up to the time of going to press, no article has been published that was able to refute the conclusions by Costa et al. There has only been unspecific criticism.

K1a1b1a spread through Europe with the migration of Jews to other European countries. The four founder lineages may be considered "Jewish" lineages, but they are not related to a Judean origin. The higher frequency of K1a1b1a among Ashkenazis may well be due to an early admixture between Judean men and European women leading to enrichment of this lineage among the relatively small Judean-European population. It is therefore logical that the frequency of K1a1b1a is much higher among Ashkenazis than among non-Jews (see also pp. 69 – 70). This relationship probably misled many population geneticists who considered the four founder lineages typical "Jewish-Middle-Eastern" based on the differences in frequency (assuming a straight relationship between Jews and Judeans). For example, Feder et al. (2007) write:

> [...] the differences between Jews and non-Jews was consistent both in the RU and Polish populations. These findings [...] support the interpretation of little or no gene flow of the local non-Jewish communities in Poland and Russia to the Jewish communities in these countries [...] consistent with the view that the ancestry of the Ashkenazic Jewish population is a result of at least four different founder events.

The differences between Thomas et al. and Behar et al. on the one side and Costa et al. on the other are also mentioned by Toch (2018, 32) who thereby refers to the New York Times: "no consensus exists yet on the 'gentile' or 'Jewish' character of female ancestry [...] the question remains moot as to whether 'many Jewish communities outside Israel were founded by single men who married and converted local women."

Another point Toch and other Jewish history scholars do not seem to realize is that we do not need a large population to convert in order to end up with a major non-Jewish lineage. In the case of a few Jewish men who came to Europe, and married women carrying a certain non-Jewish lineage, the female descendants will all have this non-Jewish lineage. If the second and maybe a few more generations continue this practice, after some time, this lineage might become a major "Jewish" lineage in the region where this took place. This is exactly what happened with K1a1b1a, for example.

The work by Costa et al. (2013) has another interesting finding: the major and most of the minor mtDNA lineages are unevenly divided between West and East European Ashkenazis. This means that there are genetic differences between West and East European Ashkenazis. In 2004, there were two publications in which a difference between West and East European Ashkenazis was also found. In the first study, pertaining to Y chromosomes, Behar et al. (2004a) showed in a multidimensional scaling (MDS) plot that German Jews were situated separately from East European Ashkenazis. In the second study, with mtDNA (Behar et al. 2004b), a genetic difference between West and East European Ashkenazis was found: only West European Ashkenazis had a genetic bottleneck. In both cases, the authors had no explanation for the difference. A genetic bottleneck is a strong reduction in genetic diversity. This happens for example when a large population is decimated as a result of war or disease, or when a small group of individuals leaves a population, moves to a different region, and "takes along" only a small part of the genetic diversity of the total population. The result of a bottleneck may be compared to that of a founder effect, as we will see on p. 53.

The conclusions by Costa et al. concerning the European origin of the three K lineages were criticized by Fernández et al. (2014). They maintain that the reason the three K lineages are not found in the Near East may be due to the loss of these lineages since Neolithic times. However, the authors have too few data to be able to come to such a conclusion, and they have no evidence that the Ashkenazic lineages are Near Eastern.

The controversial results regarding the number of founding mothers and their origin reflect the high level of admixture in Europe and the different mtDNA frequencies of West and East European Ashkenazis.

Studies with Y-chromosomal DNA

Y chromosomes are the sex chromosomes of men and are haploid. Men have an X (female sex chromosome) and a Y chromosome. Women have two X chromosomes. The Y chromosome determines the sex of the offspring in sexual reproduction. It yields an XY offspring, a male, or an XX offspring, a female. The sex chromosome of males and females cannot recombine normally. Because only men have a Y chromosome, it is possible to follow the male line. The most common method used is via the determination of single nucleotide polymorphisms (SNP). An SNP is a variation in one of the building blocks of DNA.

Ashkenazic Y-chromosomal Lineages (Y Lineages)

For the following discussion, it is important to keep in mind how complex the ethnic composition was of the Judeans who lived in the area of both kingdoms after the fall of the kingdom of Judah in 587 BCE and the beginning of the Common Era. For genetic research that tries to link modern Jews – Ashkenazic or other – to Judeans, this means that one should expect to find different lineages.

According to Behar et al. (2004a), the following lineages account for about 80 percent of Ashkenazis*:* E3b, G, J1, J2, Q, R1a, and R1b1. The authors concluded that E3b and J2 were founding lineages "because they are widespread both in AJ [Ashkenazic Jewish] populations and in Near Eastern populations, and occur at much lower frequencies in European non-Jewish populations". They consider the G and Q lineages, with similar distributions but lower frequencies, as minor Ashkenazic founding lineages. As to R1a and R1b, the authors mention that "[...] haplogroups such as R1b and R1a that predominate in European populations today [...] may also have been present in the Near East as part of the ancestral AJ gene pool." Ostrer and Skorecki (2013) refer to the work by Behar et al. (2004a) and consider E3b, G, J1, J2, and Q part of the ancestral gene pool, but R1a1 and R1b1 as European lineages. Behar et al. (2017) mention that only R1b is a European lineage. Nowadays the Ashkenazic R1a lineage is considered Middle Eastern.

Let us first look at the ancestral lineages in general. The different lineages make a common biblical arch-father virtually impossible, because the arch-father of the carriers of these lineages (most recent common ancestor – MRCA) would have lived tens of thousands of years ago. Different lineages listed as belonging to the ancestral gene pool seem to make sense. The only problem is, who were these ancestors? Do the aforementioned geneticists realize that the carriers of the lineages E3b, G, J1, J2, Q, and/or maybe R1a1 may represent Apiru, Shosu, Kenites, Midianites, Moabites, some of the seven tribes mentioned in Deuteronomy 7, Assyrians, and Edomites (all non-Israelite Judeans), and E3b also Portuguese? These five ancestral lineages may well have been the minimal number of different lineages among the different Judean populations. If they belonged to "converted" members of one of the non-Israelite Judeans there may not be any close genetic relationship to the Israelite Judeans. It is a bit naïve to suppose that a Middle Eastern origin automatically means an Israelite Judean background. The fact that two lineages were the most widespread among the Ashkenazic population in Europe may well be the result of the number of Judeans/Jews with these lineages who came to Europe. If the number of Judeans/Jews was relatively large, they may have become the most widespread in Europe, without being so in their homeland. A similar argument may be used against the conclusion that some are minor lineages. If these lineages were the most widespread among the Judeans in Palestine and, as it so happened, only few men with these lineages came to Europe, their lower frequencies in Europe may not be a reflection of the situation in the homeland either.

The different lineages in the ancestral gene pool have different origins as well. The expansion of the E lineage probably started in eastern Africa about 58,000 years ago (Trombetta et al. 2015). The G lineage originated most likely in the Caucasus (Rootsi et al. 2012). The authors report the highest frequency, more than 70 percent, in North Ossetians. J1 and J2 are two major sublineages of the J-M304 lineage. It is not clear where J1-M267 arose. J1-M267*(xP58), which is J1-M267 without the J-P58 lineages, has its highest frequency in the Caucasus (Balanovsky et al. 2011) while the P58 lineages have their highest frequency in the Arabian Peninsula (Chiaroni et al. 2010). J2-M172 probably arose in Anatolia (Cinnioglu et al. 2004). Q originated in Central Asia, in the Altai Mountains (Zegura et al. 2004). These different lineages are not exactly encouraging for the idea that the Israelite Judeans were a somewhat homogeneous population. The possibility that early Israelites were maybe descendants of Apiru and Shosu, and that later on their descendants intermarried with the different tribes mentioned on p. 15, would not be contradictory to these different regions of origin. The different lineages of the ancestral gene pool also agree with the 12 tribes being a metaphor for the ethnic heterogeneity of the Israelite population as suggested in chapter 1 (p. 12).

In addition to the study of Jewish men in general, studies were made of two special groups of Jews, priests and Levites.

Jewish Priests (Hebrew: כהנים – *kohanim*)

Skorecki et al. (1997) showed that Jewish priests had a specific lineage, the *Cohen modal haplotype* (CMH). The article was big news and was mentioned in one of the most widely-read national Dutch newspapers.

Still, some comments are in place. One may assume that during the diaspora, many "foreign" Y chromosomes entered the Jewish communities (especially because Jewishness is determined by the mother) that did not enter the priestly families, because a non-Jew cannot become a priest. This may also explain the difference in the composition of the Y chromosome populations of priests and lay-Jews (not mentioned by the authors). Skorecki et al. maintain that the Ashkenazic and Sephardic communities are genetically different, based on the findings by Motulsky (1995). But a statistical analysis of their data shows that there is no significant difference ($X^2 = 4.05$; 0.50<P,0.90) between the haplotypes of the Ashkenazic and Sephardic populations. One would expect no genetic difference between Ashkenazic and Sephardic priests, as no non-Jew can become a priest, and the priests are supposed to be a clearly defined group. A genetic difference would be expected between Ashkenazic and Sephardic lay-Jews. However, exactly the opposite was found. The final blow to the article was given by Zoossmann-Diskin (2000) who showed two things: firstly, that the lineage occurred in non-Jewish populations as well; and secondly, that "the way the authors define the term 'Sephardic' is probably related to its use in Israeli religious politics; it has nothing to do with science." This term should only be used for descendants of Iberian Jews, and not for North African (ibid.) and Turkish Jews (see also my comment in *Plos One* on the article by Behar et al. (2008) in chapter 6). The article by Zoossmann-Diskin has not been referred to in the English genetic literature.

More information has become available that indicates that Jewish priests, like lay-Judeans, could have different genetic backgrounds. According to Talmon (2005, 455), King Jeroboam I (Hebrew: ירבעם; reigned at the end of the tenth century BCE), re-established

> the ancient cult places in Bethel and Dan (1 Kings 12:28; 13:32) as rival shrines of the Temple of Jerusalem and the installation there of priests of his own choice from the 'elite of the people' מקצות העם (1 Kings 12:31–32; 13:33), whom the Chronicler disparagingly designates 'priests from the (common) people' כהנים בעמי הארצות (2 Chronicles 13:8–9).

Thus, the king could appoint anyone he liked to become a priest. This was clearly contrary to religious tradition, but it may be another explanation of the different lineages among priests.

Well over 10 years after the article by Skorecki et al. (1997), Hammer et al. (2009) admitted that the CMH was not an old priestly haplotype, without referring to Zoossmann-Diskin's article. They found 21 lineages among priests. The two most frequent CMHs are J1e*-P58* and an extended CMH (eCMH) J2a-M410*, carried by 46 and 14 percent of the Jewish priests, respectively, that have their origin in the Middle East. A coalescence analysis for lay-Jews and priests with J-P58* resulted in a TMRCA of 4,415 years. The lineages with frequencies greater than 5 percent were J2-M12, J2-M318, and R-M269 with 7.4, 6.1, and 5.6

percent, respectively. In addition to lineage R, lineage E was also among the rare lineages.

The simple fact that they found 21 different lineages among priests, belonging to at least three different haplogroups (J, R, and E) makes a single origin even for priests virtually impossible. One of the models Hammer et al. suggest to explain the various lineages is a metapopulation "in which semi-isolated communities maintain multiple Cohen lineages". I assume that the model operates within the Judean environment. There is a possibility though that some of the Jewish priests may have a Middle Eastern origin, but not related to the "official" priests as recognized by the kingdom of Judah: namely, a non-related Canaanite priestly family, appointed by the abovementioned King Jeroboam I. Haber et al. (2017) investigated ancient DNA (aDNA) from five Bronze Age individuals who lived in Sidon some 3700 years ago. Sidon was a Canaanite city. They found two individuals with Y lineages, J1-P58 and J2-M12, respectively. These lineages are also carried by modern Jewish priests (Hammer et al. 2009). As mentioned before, King Ahab of the northern kingdom married a Phoenician princess (p. 17), and the rural population in the north consisted also of Phoenicians (p. 14). In 2008, Zalloua et al. reported that J2 was a Phoenician associated lineage. It would be interesting to find out what the relationship is between modern Jewish priests with J1-P58 and J2-M12 and the Phoenicians (i.e. Canaanites) who had converted. These Canaanites and the priests with J1-P58 and J2-M12 may have been genetically similar. What about the other lineages mentioned, could there be a link with, for example, Arameans, Moabites, or Midianites? As we saw before, Moses married the daughter of a Midianite priest. If some of the other lineages were carried by the 3 tribes just mentioned, does that mean that they were considered part of the 12 tribes?

If we just look at the J1 and J2 lineages in general, the two most common ones among Jewish priests, both belonging to lineage J, we have a similar problem as with the lay-Jews: according to the biblical history, Aaron, the forefather of Jewish priests, lived about 3,300 years ago, which implies that the split of the J lineage into J1 and J2 must have occurred after that time. However, the split into J1 and J2 took place more than 25,000 years ago (Finocchio 2018, Supplemental Figure 4). Taking into account that a king could appoint a priest from "the elite of the people", without specifying whom he considered "the elite", it is not clear what the ethnic background of such a priest may have been. With the multi-ethnic population of the northern kingdom, it is thus impossible to know to what ethnic group the carrier of the abovementioned lineages belonged.

Moreover, the finding that the J1 and J2 lineages are the most frequent ones among Ashkenazic priests, may just be the result of the number of persons with these lineages moving to Europe from the Middle East, similar to the explanation of the most frequent lineages among lay-Jews. That being the case, the difference between Ashkenazic and Sephardic priests may well have been due to the particular lineage a priest belonged to when he came to Spain or the "Ashkenazic" part of Europe. The finding of a modal haplotype for Ashkenazic priests does not mean anything as to its modality in the Land of Israel, as long as we do not know what the frequency was of the priests with this lineage before they came to Europe. If by chance, most of the priests who came to Europe carried a lineage that was a minor lineage in the Middle East, geneticists who study Ashkenazic priests, may well consider this lineage as indicative of the original Judean priests. How justified is this conclusion? We are not even sure that his forefather was a priest according to the official view of the kingdom of Judah. We do not know what lineage the majority of the original priests carried, or if there was such a majority. And what is the status of the less frequent lineages mentioned by Hammer et al.? As long as today's Jewish priests carry several different lineages, it is pretty clear that there wasn't one forefather, and it also remains unclear what the relationship is between the "official" biblical priests and today's priests.

Levites

The hypothesis that Levites have one forefather is just as problematic as it is for the lay-Jews and the priests. The heterogeneous origin of Levites has been suggested by a number of geneticists (Thomas et al. 1998; Bradman et al. 2000, 35; Behar et al. 2003), indicating that Levites are not descendants of one tribal group either. The results of Thomas and Bradman do not indicate that non-Jewish groups are involved as ancestors. On the other hand, Behar et al. found that European haplotype R1a1 was present in more than 50 percent of Ashkenazic Levites. Although I discussed their article in an earlier publication (van Straten 2011a, 151–154), there is another problem that should be mentioned. The article also shows what happens when wrong historical/demographic assumptions are made with regards to sampling the individuals. Of the 60 Levites sampled, 65 percent came from Central and Eastern Europe. The remaining 35 percent came from Germany, Netherlands, and France. As no genealogical research was carried out as to a possible East European ancestry of the 35 percent, it is not certain to what extent Jews from the last three countries were really West European. The authors sampled three non-Jewish populations "because of their geographic location relative to the ancestral European communities of Ashkenazic Jews [...]": Germans, Sorbians, and Belarusians. They also added a Norwegian group because "it represented a geographic location that excluded Jewish entry until the middle of the 19th century [...]".

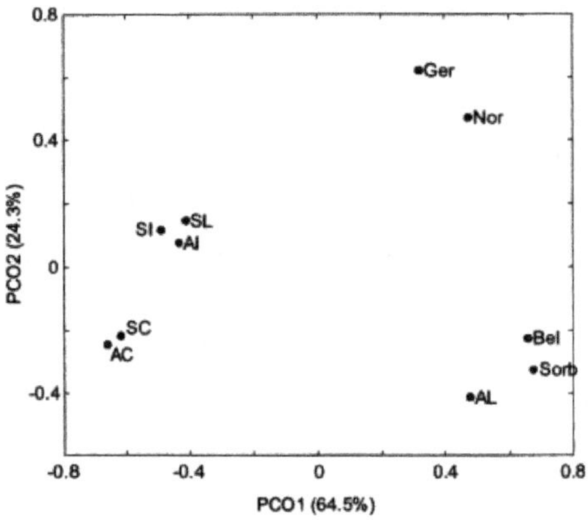

Figure 4: The principal coordinates plot derived from the genetic similarity values (Behar et al. (2003).

In their principal coordinates plot (Figure 4) they found an "unusual distribution of Ashkenazic Levite (AL) haplogroup frequencies". The Ashkenazic Levites clustered relatively close to Belarusians (Bel) and Sorbians (Sorb), as seen on the lower right part of the figure, and not with the other Jewish groups. The latter two clustered close to each other. However, the Germans (Ger) clustered close to the Norwegians (Nor), as seen on the top right of the figure, far away from the Levites. Germans appeared to be no more related to the Ashkenazic Levites than the Norwegians. This was not expected, because the authors think that Ashkenazis originate from Germany, and thus expected admixture. However, there is no evidence for a German origin, and most of the Levites in the study were East Europeans. Therefore, the clustering of Germans and Norwegians in this plot makes sense, and Germans should not have been included with the Sorbians and Belarusians. Nebel et al. (2005) report that European R1a1 (R-M17) lineage, present at high frequencies in Ukrainians, Belarusians, Poles, and Hungarians (average frequency: 55 percent), was also found among the general Ashkenazic population with a frequency of 11.5 percent. Irrespective of the question from which European population R-M17 entered the Jewish population, the presence of this lineage is controversial as it is against the Jewish law that non-Jews can become Levites.

As we saw before, Ostrer and Skorecki (2013) consider R1a and R1b as European lineages, while Behar et al. (2017) consider only R1b as European, and R1a as a Levite lineage. But R1a is a completely different lineage from those of the ancestral gene pool. This is strange, because Levites should be part of the total ancestral gene pool as well.

In 2013, Rootsi et al. refuted the conclusions by Behar et al. about the Levites. Due to the fractionation of R1a, the R1a-M582 lineage was discovered with a high frequency among Ashkenazic Levites (65 percent within the Jewish castes), and with very low percentages among the priests and laymen. The percentage R1a-M582 among non-Ashkenazic Levites was lower, only 8 percent. The most common recent ancestor lived between 1500 and 2500 years ago. The lineage originated in the Middle East, was almost absent among non-Jewish Europeans, and was brought to Europe by Jewish migrants.

Levites always formed a small percentage of the Judeans or Jews. An estimate of 4 percent among Ashkenazis (Bradman et al. 2000, 33) is a rough guess. It is based on an unpublished undergraduate project by Bradman in 1996. He surveyed 400 graves of Ashkenazic and Sephardic Jews in London, and found that about 4 percent of the men were Levites. How representative is this percentage for Ashkenazis in general? Nebel et al. (2005) found 11.5 percent for Ashkenazic Jewry. They report a range from 0.25 to 3.4 percent (Kosmin and Waterman 1989, and DellaPergola 1984, respectively). The 0.25 percent however, refers to the percentage of Jews among people with the surname Levy (personal communication by Kosmin). DellaPergola writes that 3.4 percent of the Italian Jews bear the name Levi. This does not mean that they are Levites. Nebel at al. (2005) also report that Passarino et al. (2001) found 9.7 percent Levites for Ashkenazic Jewry. However, Passarino et al. do not mention Levites, only Ashkenazis. They took their data from Santachiara Benerecetti et al. (1993) who only write about Ashkenazi Jews. The lineage in question is Eu19/49a,f Ht11 (R-M17) that emerged in Ukraine There may be many reasons for the wide range:

1. There is no information about the size of the different tribes, during biblical times, including the Levites. This means that we have no information about the percentage of Levites of the total Judean population.
2. We do not know the background of the people who called themselves Levites.
3. The genetic background of the original Levites is unknown.
4. There is no knowledge about how many Levites came to Europe, not in absolute terms, but also not relative to the number of lay-Jews. Similarly, we do not know how many Levites went where in Europe.
5. There is not always a connection between the surname Levy and the Levite cast.
6. The difference between Ashkenazic and non-Ashkenazic Levites may, similar to the situation of the priests, be due to the specific lineage the Levite carried when he went to Ashkenazic Europe or somewhere else.

All these points make it difficult to determine the percentage of Levites in the Ashkenazic or other Jewish population. It may be assumed though that the number of Levites who came to Europe was small compared to the lay-Jews. With few Levites coming to Europe, it is also not out of the ordinary that one finds mainly one lineage among Ashkenazic Levites. Actually, we see here the same arguments used to explain the percentage of Levites among Ashkenazis as those used to explain the percentage of priests. Thus, the fact that R1a-M582 occurred with a frequency of 65 percent may well be the result of the number of Levites who came to Europe, and who just happened to carry this lineage, without it being the modal lineage of the Levites in the Land of Israel. Furthermore, the fact that R1a-M582 originated in the Middle East is (again) no proof that the "original" Levites had R1a-M582. Finally, there should be a common lineage of Levites and lay-Jews (and priests) some 4000 years ago, but there isn't one.

In their discussion of the genetic variation among Levites, Behar et al. (2017) write: "According to the Biblical narrative [...] Levi was the third son of [...] Jacob [...] one great-grandson of Levi, named Aaron [...] the first high priest." As there was also no one forefather of the Levites, it does not make sense to quote the Bible in this case. The article by Behar et al. (2017) has another questionable point. In their Figure 1, they show the expansion of the Ashkenazic Levite Y chromosome lineage into Europe via Italy and also via Girona, Catalonia, Spain. The route via Girona is based on the genealogical history of the Horowitz family. To use family history in a scientific paper is rather tricky. We have a lot of genealogical experience in Amsterdam, thanks to the extant registrations of the Jewish community, starting in the seventeenth century and the beginning of the eighteenth century, for example, the buying and selling of seats in the Great Synagogue, burial books, circumcisions, marriage contracts (Hebrew: *tena'im aharonim*), and marriage certificates (Hebrew: *ketubot*). We also have experience with Jews coming to the Netherlands from far-away countries. When the immigrant came from far, he/she normally went to a big city, as it was most likely that there were other Jews who could understand him/her here. The possibilities for trade were greater there as well. This holds also for the Iberian Jews. They came to cities like Amsterdam and The Hague (Antwerp, Belgium and Hamburg, Germany). In the countryside, we normally find Jews from Germany, our eastern neighbor. There is an interesting phenomenon in the Netherlands that should be mentioned when the discussion is about Ashkenazic and Sephardic Jews. A number of Ashkenazis try to show by all means that they are actually descendants of Sephardic Jews. The Sephardic Jews were the elite with money and influence, while Ashkenazic ancestors were mostly poor people. Sephardic ancestry gives social status (at least that is what some people think). With this background, let us go back to the Horowitz family.

Before trying to find out something about the Horowitz family, I already had some doubts about the story. The migration of a Sephardic rabbi from a big city like Girona to a small place with an Ashkenazic community like Hořovice is not very likely. Spanish rabbis spoke Spanish, not Czech, German, or Yiddish. There were also religious differences between Sephardic and Ashkenazic Jews. For example, Sephardic Jews are allowed to eat legumes on Passover, while Ashkenazis are not. The levirate marriage (Deuteronomy 25: 5–10; man marries his brother's widow) was practically annulled in the Ashkenazic community, while it was enforced in the Sephardic community (Ta-Shma 2003, 58). How would the Ashkenazic community of Hořovice have reacted to a Sephardic rabbi with his different customs? Hardly any Jew from Iberia went to Bohemia and Moravia, or Eastern Europe for that matter. According to Avraham (2010), "Sephardic Jews were a marginal element in Eastern Europe [...] Jews expelled from the Iberian Peninsula at the end of the fifteenth century, and *conversos* leaving those lands in later periods, did not settle in Eastern Europe." Finally, Sephardic Jews who came to France, Belgium, England, Germany, and the Netherlands, kept their Iberian surnames. Why would a Spanish rabbi change his Iberian surname to that of a relatively unknown small town in Bohemia?

However, there is also solid evidence that the Girona connection was made up in the nineteenth century. Marmorstein (2016) discussed the question of whether the Horowitz family descends from the Benvenisti ha-levi family from Spain. The discussion is a review of publications between 1701 and 2004 about the family tree of the Horowitz family. He shows a copy of the earliest history of the Horowitz family written by rabbi Shabtai ha-levi Horowitz (1590–1660) that was added to a book published in Amsterdam in 1701, entitled *sefer yesh nohalin* (there are heirs; Horowitz 1701), written by his grandfather Avraham Horowitz (1540–1615). I checked the source, and Figures 5 and 6 show a picture of the title page and the page with the family history, respectively. The latter is found in the first section on the right.

The earliest forefather in the will is Yeshaya. Exactly as Marmorstein writes, no mention is made of an Iberian connection. It is very unlikely that Shabtai ha-levi would not have been informed about an origin from Spain if it involved a well-known rabbi. Marmorstein shows that also in the next family history of the Horowitz family in 1740, no mention is made of Iberia. I will only mention two more publications Marmorstein refers to. Horowitz (1931) summarizes his family history, based on the family history printed in his father's book *haye arye* (the life of Arye) as follows (translated from German):

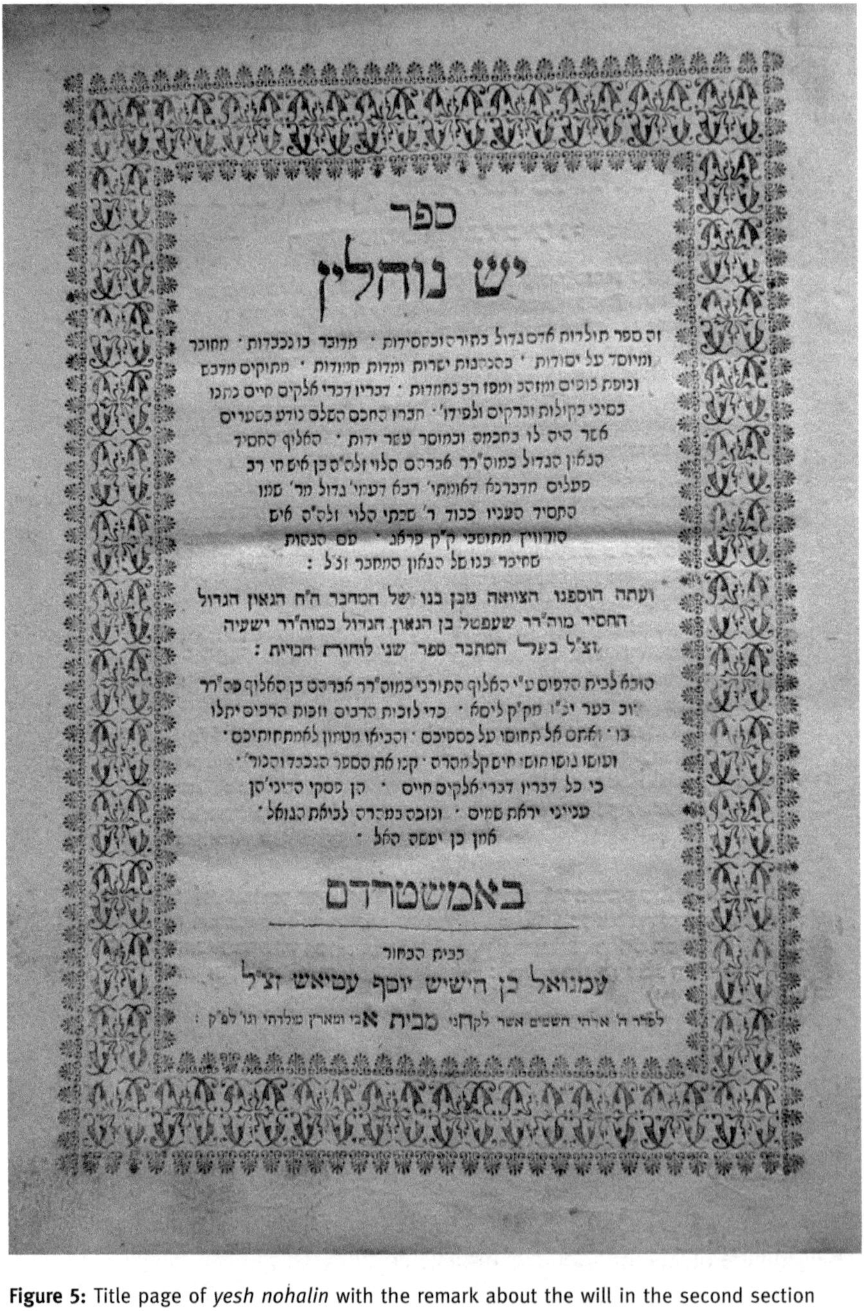

ספר
יש נוחלין
זה ספר תולדות אדם גדול בתורה ובחסידות · מדובר בו נכבדות · מחובר
ומיוסד על יסודות · בהנהגות ישרות ומדות חמודות · מתוקים מדבש
ונופת צופים ומזהב ומפז רב נחמדות · דבריו דברי אלקים חיים נתנו
בסיני בקולות וברקים ולפידו' · חברו החכם השלם נודע בשערים
אשר היה לו בחכמה ובמוסר עשר ידות · האלוף החסיד
הגאון הגדול כמוה"רר אברהם הלוי זלה"ה בן איש חי רב
פעלים מדברנא דאומתי' רבא דעמי' גדול מר' שמו
החסיד העניו כבוד ר' שבתי הלוי זלה"ה איש
הורוויץ מתושבי ק"ק פראג · עם הגהות
שחיבר בנו של הגאון המחבר ז"ל :

ועתה הוספנו הצוואה מבן בנו של המחבר ה"ח הגאון הגדול
החסיד מוה"רר שעפטל בן הגאון הגדול כמוה"רר ישעיה
זצ"ל בעל המחבר ספר שני לוחות הברית :

הובא לבית הדפוס ע"י האלוף התורני כמוה"רר אברהם בן האלוף כה"רר
יוב בער יצ"ו מק"ק ליסא · כדי לזכות הרבים וזכות הרבים יתלו
בו · ואתם אל תחוסו על כספיכם · והביאו מטמון לאמתחותיכם ·
ועוסו נוסו חוסו חיש קל מהרה · קנו את הספר הנכבד והנזכר ·
כי כל דבריו דברי אלקים חיים · הן פסקי דינים הן
ענייני יראת שמים · ונזכה במהרה לביאת הגואל ·
אמן כן יעשה האל ·

באמשטרדם

בבית הבחור
עמנואל בן הישיש יוסף עטיאש זצ"ל
לסדר ה' אלהי השמים אשר לקחני מבית אבי ומארץ מולדתי וגו' לפ"ק :

Figure 5: Title page of *yesh nohalin* with the remark about the will in the second section (Bibliotheca Rosenthaliana, University of Amsterdam).

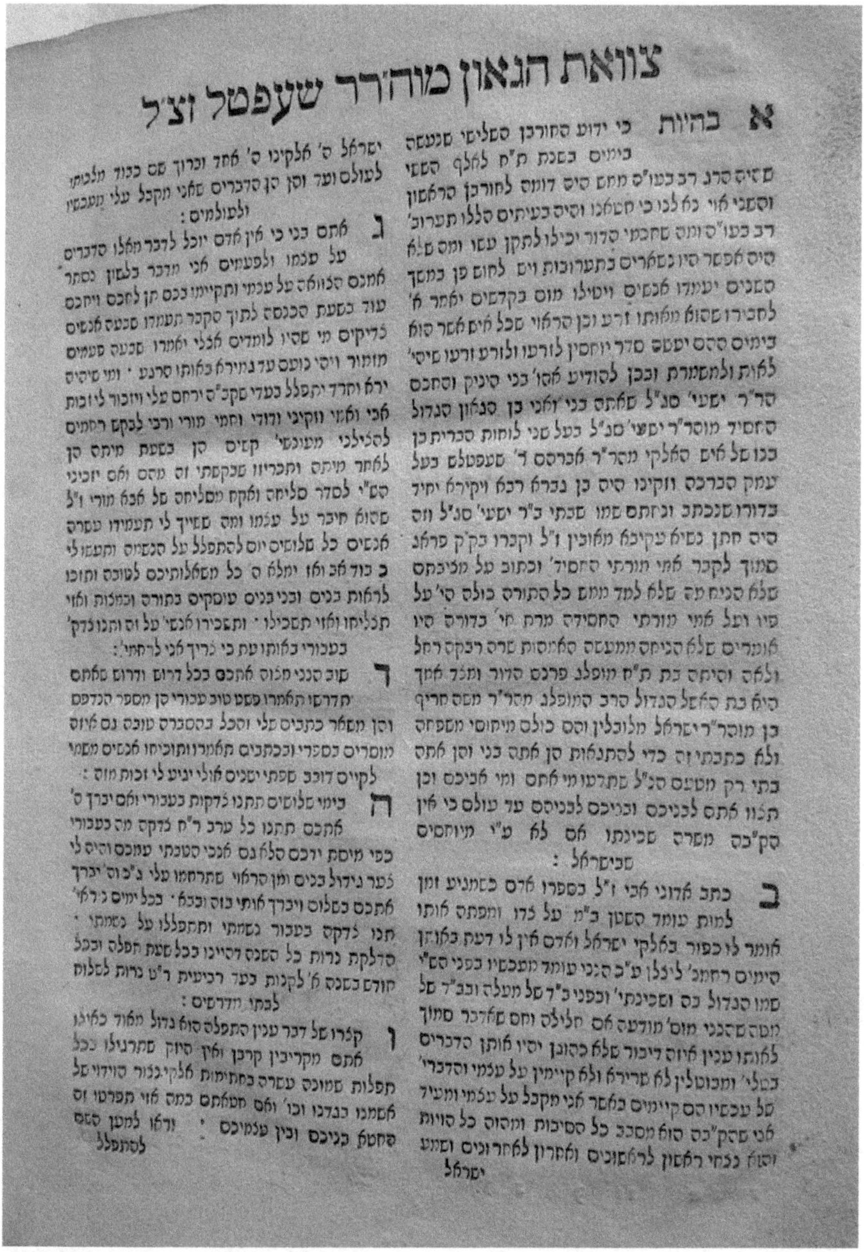

Figure 6: The ethical will of rabbi Shabtai halevi Horowitz (1590 – 1660) in the first section on the right (Bibliotheca Rosenthaliana, University of Amsterdam).

> According to the tradition, the Horowitz family originates from Spain as descendants of R. Isaak ha-Levy, whose father R. Pinchas ha-Levy, brother of the famous R. Aaron ha-Levy הר"אה, originated from Barcelona. The latter were sons of R. Josef ha-Levy, son of the famous R. Serachja ha-Levy [...] who was the son of R. Isaak ha-Levy of Gerona and grandson of R. Schem Tauw ha-Levy, who lived in the 11th century. According to tradition, they are descendants of the prophet Samuel, a descendant of Jizhar, son of Kehoss ben Levy, son of arch-father and patriarch Jakob.

After mentioning that a member of the family moved to Bohemia as a result of a pogrom in Spain, "maybe in 1390", Horowitz writes (translated from German): "he bought the country estate "Horowitz" not far from Prague, and therefore was called the man from Horowitz איש הורוויץ (*ish horowits*)." The inclusion of a legend in the family history is not really an addition to make it more reliable, and the remaining part of the family tree therefore also becomes questionable, especially since Shabtai ha-levi Horowitz seems to be ignorant of all these ancestors. Furthermore, it is generally assumed that the name Horowitz comes from the town Hořovice. The inclusion of the prophet is interesting. It shows how legends become part of genealogy. R. Aharon and his ancestors signed as היצהרי (*ha-yitshari*, descendant of Yitshar) or sometimes as הקהתי (*ha-kehati*, descendant of Kehat), who were a son and grandson respectively of Levi son of arch father Jacob (Rotner 2004). The claim that these rabbis, and thus the Horowitz family, descend from the prophet comes from Shmelke Horowitz (7 generations after Yeshaya) who declared at his death that the prophet Samuel was one of the descendants of Yitshar son of Kehat, son of Levi (ibid.). It should be noted that Rotner does not make a critical remark about the family tree back to Samuel or earlier.

At the end of his article, Marmorstein (2016) writes:

> One wonders whether – given the fact that a devoted genealogist of the family [Shabtai halevi Horowitz] living in the 1740's [sic] had not heard of a connection to the illustrious ancestor Rabbi Zerachya Halevi and the Benvenisti Family – this family documented 140 years later should be considered reliable? [...] Perhaps we should consider it more of a tradition and legend than an established fact [...].

Why then does the Horowitz family originate all of a sudden from Girona in 1883? I can only refer to the status aspect mentioned above. Maybe it gives more status to be a descendant of a famous Sephardic rabbi from Spain than to be a descendant of a rabbi from Hořovice. Whatever the reason, the authors of the DNA article should have checked the sources for their information more carefully. A large part of the work could have been avoided, and a large part of this discussion could have been omitted. Of course, it looks nice to include a well-known Sephardic rabbi in the genetic investigation, but not in such an amateurish way.

A somewhat curious point in the article by Behar et al. (2017) is a reference to Leuchter's book, *Levites and boundaries of Israelite identity.* The authors only mention that "Alternative theories for the origins of the Levite caste have been proposed" without informing the reader about what these theories might be. According to Leuchter (2017, 92), the early priests were descendants of Moses, the Mushites, in the twelfth century BCE: "It is around these priestly lineages that the Levite caste was built, drawn from lay families devoted to the sanctuaries where priestly clans like the Mushites dominated." Such recruitment could possibly lead to different lineages among the Levites as well. However, they should still be similar to one of the lineages of the lay-Jews if the Bible story is correct.

One might consider it irrelevant to even mention the Bible story, but for some the biblical history plays an important role in Jewish history. It should be mentioned though that the archeological findings do not substantiate the Hebrew Bible as a historical document either.

Reason for the controversial results of all three groups – lay-Jews, priests, and Levites – is the idea that one can explain the origin of a population defined by religion via genetics. The rabbinical ruling makes this impossible, irrespective of the biblical history. Without mentioning the rabbinical ruling, Falk (2017, 208) rightfully writes "[...] there is no proof of a typical Jewish prototype. Biology alone cannot provide proof to identify Jews as such. There are no Jewish genes [...]." On the other hand, the genetic results are not controversial with regards to the rabbinical definition of a Jew, at least not for the overwhelming majority of lay-Jews, because the definition includes converts.

Demographic Data and Uniparental Markers

Uniparental markers are markers on the DNA that are typical for one of the parents: on mtDNA (the mother) and Y chromosomes (the father).

In a reaction against the idea that Y-chromosomal lineages point to a Middle Eastern origin of East European Jews, Zoossmann-Diskin (2010) writes:

> [this] is erroneous not only because the Y-chromosomal analysis contradicts the analyses based on the other chromosomes, and because the NRY [non-recombining region of the Y chromosome] is a single uniparental marker that does not represent the whole history of the population [...] The demographic histories [...] exemplify how different demographic patterns make the uniparental markers more reliable for Iraqi (Babylonian) Jews and Yemenite Jews and less reliable for EEJ [East European Jews].

He provides the following demographic history about the Yemenite Jews: “Yemenite Jews [...] were numerous enough to have an independent kingdom in the first centuries AD [...] They numbered a few hundred thousand in the 12th century AD, and gradually declined; reaching only about 30 – 40,000 at the beginning of the 20th century”.

The sentence about the kingdom is somewhat misleading because the Himyarite kingdom is meant as consisting mostly of Yemenites who converted to Judaism. The kingdom did not last long, and eventually most of the converts converted to Islam. The number of a few hundred thousand is not reliable either (personal communication by Yosef Tobi of the University of Haifa). Zoossmann-Diskin gives the following sizes of the Jewish population in Iraq: more than a million Jews in the first century CE, 806,000 by 600 CE, about one million in the seventh century, and 70,000 to hundreds of thousands in the fourteenth century. Considering that from the beginning of the Common Era up to 600 CE the population of Iraq stayed constant at about 1 million (McEvedy and Jones 1978, 151), the sizes of the Jewish population are not realistic. As to the situation in the fourteenth century, the hundreds of thousands are mentioned by Arab writers of whom Sassoon (1949, 7, 89, 103), the author who provides the numbers, says that this number is not dependable. The number of 70,000 is for the year 1308 Hijrah (Islam calendar), or 1890 – 1891 CE, and has nothing to do with the fourteenth century CE. As to East European Jews, Zoossmann-Diskin mentions the “out of Germany” line with its high annual growth rates and the East European Jewish population of the Polish-Lithuanian Commonwealth who went through the opposite process: “Their history is one of founder effects, migrations, demographic bottlenecks and finally a rapid expansion.” Thus, there is also a flaw in this demographic history.

We see here that wrong demographic data about Yemenite and Iraqi Jews are used to show that these Jews went through a demographic development that was opposite to that of East European Jews of whom the demographic history is not correct either. Thus, these demographic histories do not exemplify anything. The author may be right about the use of uniparental markers, but his rebuttal of the assumption that the Y chromosomes of East European Ashkenazis point to a Middle Eastern origin is based on three erroneous demographic histories.

Studies with Autosomal DNA

Development of a Population-genetic Test based on Demographic Data

Slatkin developed a population-genetic test of the founder effect hypothesis as related to Ashkenazic Jewish diseases, based on demographic data. A founder effect is a term used in population genetics to denote a situation whereby a few people leave a large population and found a new population. In such a case, there will be a loss of genetic information, because the few people only carry part of the genetic information of the large population.

In the introduction, the author refers to a founding in 750 and in 1700 CE, in Germany and Lithuania respectively. However, these Jewish population centers were not founded in these years. Both were founded hundreds of years earlier. In addition, the former refers to Ashkenazis by descent (German Jews), while the latter refers to Ashkenazis by rites (East European Jews).

Further on, he writes the following:

> Although current uncertainty about the early demographic history of the AJ [Ashkenazic Jewish] population will not allow a strong conclusion to be reached, the results show that the available genetic data for AJ disease alleles are consistent with the founder-effect hypothesis if plausible assumptions are made about early AJ population sizes.

Let us look at the plausible assumptions about the Jewish population sizes. I will only show Slatkin's population sizes between 1096 and 1765 (Table 3). The number of 150,000 in 1096 is supposedly taken from Engelman, but I did not find this number in his publication. Engelman (1960) does write though that by the end of the fifteenth century there were probably fewer than 300,000 Jews on the entire European continent. He does not show how he arrived at this number, and there is no factual evidence for it either. Furthermore, the population sizes in Table 3 are based on the data by Baron, Weinryb and DellaPergola, which I showed in chapter 2 to be implausible. The growth rates in Table 3 are not plausible.

In Slatkin's article, we are confronted again with the problem of mixing up Ashkenazis by descent (German Jews) and Ashkenazis almost only according to rites (East European Ashkenazis). The conclusion by Slatkin, that "the available genetic data for AJ disease alleles are consistent with the founder effect hypothesis", is not based on plausible demographic assumptions.

Table 3: Jewish population sizes in different years with corresponding annual growth rates according to Slatkin (2004).

Year		Annual growth rate %
1096	150,000	
1348	600 – 6,000	
		2.1 – 0.6
1500	15,000	
		1.8
1648	200,000	
		Negative growth
1667	16,0000	
		1.6
1765	750,000	

Four Jewish Grandparents as Proof of a Middle Eastern Origin

Need et al. (2009) assessed whether self-identified (Ashkenazic) Jewish ancestry can be inferred from genomic information from individuals with four or fewer Jewish grandparents. They used PCA, whereby about 550,000 polymorphic markers were used per individual. The authors collected a random sample of 611 Caucasian subjects, mostly residing in America. The number of Jewish grandparents varied from zero to four. They found that individuals with full Jewish ancestry formed a clearly distinct cluster from those with no Jewish ancestry. One individual with four Jewish grandparents, who did not know the country of origin of the grandparents, was intermediate between the two clusters. The individuals with fewer than four Jewish grandparents were intermediate between the two clusters as well. When the Jewish individuals were compared with non-Jewish individuals from the Middle East and Europe, the Jewish cluster was located approximately midway between the clusters of the two aforementioned groups. The authors concluded that the distinction from non-Jewish Europeans is more due to genetic heritage in the Middle East than to bottlenecks, with possible inbreeding.

Given the problems with the studies discussed so far, the extent of early admixture, and the resulting phenotypical resemblance of Ashkenazis with non-Jewish Europeans, the conclusion of Need et al. seems questionable. Another questionable point is the definition of pure Jews: four Jewish grandparents. From genealogy, it is known that people may have some detailed information about their grandparents, but it is unusual that they have such information about earlier generations. Thanks to extant Hebrew burial books of the Jewish community of Amsterdam (1669 – 1811), we know that 119 of the dead were converts (van Straten 2009, 159). Without such records, who would know about his or her converted ancestor? It can be virtually excluded that the subjects sampled by Need et al. knew anything about their ancestors in Eastern Europe from the eighteenth century or earlier, a large percentage did not even know details about their grandparents. Because of substantial admixture, especially during the first millennium CE, as known from historical data, and especially as shown recently, it is questionable if four Jewish grandparents mean anything as to a Middle Eastern origin. All it means is that the four grandparents were (East European) Ashkenazis as well (or had converted to Judaism). The following quote emphasizes the unfamiliarity of many geneticists with the extent of admixture during the first millennium and earlier: "Our conclusion favoring common ancestry over recent admixture is further supported by the fact that our sample contains individuals that are known not to be admixed in the most recent one or two generations" (Behar et al. 2010). Because the definition of Jews also implies converts, it may not even be possible to speak of genetically pure Jews, but only of religiously pure Jews.

There are thus a number of important drawbacks to the work of Need et al., and I would like to propose that the differences between the clusters are due to geographic differences and not to "Jewishness". Let us, therefore, take a closer look at the raw data of the two main groups, the subjects with four Jewish grandparents, and the subjects with no Jewish grandparents. It appears that within the known countries of origin, 85 percent of the maternal grandparents and 74 percent of the paternal grandparents came from Eastern Europe. This is in agreement with earlier findings (Lestschinsky 1960, 1536 – 1596). It should be mentioned that it was unknown where 47 percent of the grandparents came from. This is only two generations ago. It is unlikely that the picture would be changed significantly if the origin of this 47 percent would be known. Guha et al. (2012) used the same cohort of Ashkenazis as Need et al. did in their study to show that pooling West and East European Ashkenazis was legitimate. However, as we just saw, these Ashkenazis were virtually all East European. Therefore, the legitimacy of the pooling procedure becomes questionable.

The situation among the non-Jewish grandparents is a bit less clear. About 90 percent of Caucasian non-Jewish Americans originate from Northern Europe, Western Europe, Austria, and Southern Europe (Farley and Haaga 2005; Department of Justice, immigration and naturalization service 2007). Need et al. reported that within the known regions of origin, Northwestern and Southern Europe provide 80 percent of the grandparents. Again, there is a clear preference for one part of Europe: Northwestern Europe. The 80 percent is somewhat lower than the

90 percent mentioned above, but it should be noticed that an even higher percentage, 69 percent, of the country of origin of the grandparents was unknown.

East European Jews have a genetic make-up between that of South Europeans and Middle Easterners with some genetic inflow from East Europeans. A difference between East European Jews and Northwest Europeans would be a better explanation for the difference between the clusters than a difference between Jews and non-Jews. It would explain the substantial admixture (Costa et al. 2013; Carmi et al. 2014; Behar et al. 2004a), the related European physical appearance (phenotype), and it would agree with the U.S. immigration data (Lestschinsky 1960, 1536–1596).

The Use of a Model to Determine the Size of a Genetic Bottleneck

Palamara et al. (2012) looked at different models from which they chose the one that resulted in the right demographic history of Ashkenazic Jewry as part of their methodology. They obtained a genetic bottleneck of 270 Ashkenazis (effective population size) around 1150. An effective population size describes the number of people in an idealized population that under certain circumstances would be equal to the number of people in the real or census population. The effective population size is normally smaller than the census population size. The effective population size of Ashkenazis is not far from one-third of the census population size (Cavalli-Sforza and Carmelli 1979, 97). This would give a census population size of about 800. With 2.22 million East European, German, and Dutch Ashkenazis in 1800 (I did not collect numerical data about other Ashkenazis), the resulting annual growth rate is 1.2 percent over 650 years. It is obvious that such a growth rate is unlikely during this period. One of the models they did not choose resulted in "unrealistically large values for the recent population size". Normally when one finds a population size x at t_1, and the population size y at t_2 is known, and in this case it is known, one calculates the annual growth rate. It cannot be that a known population size at t_2 appears that is too large. This means that the criterion for accepting the model is not correct. In the introduction, the authors write: "We analyzed a cohort of Ashkenazi Jewish (AJ) individuals by reconstructing a strong founder event [...] in agreement with historical accounts." The authors matched the numbers they got with what they considered to be the best candidate events in history books, the migration east. This is exactly the problem because there was no migration east (except by some individuals), and it is also this migration that would have been responsible for the implausible growth rates. The model referred to clearly had a much larger bottleneck size. The authors should have determined the growth rate of this larger population size to reach the roughly 2.2 million Ashkenazis in 1800 in order to evaluate the validity of their model. What we see here is that a wrong model was chosen, due to a wrong assumption, namely the migration east with its demographic implications.

In a second study, a bottleneck was calculated with 350 Ashkenazis 700 years ago resulting in an annual growth rate of 1.8 percent (Carmi et al. 2014). This growth rate is even less plausible in Europe during this period. In Eastern Europe alone in 1400, there were between 306,000 and 544,500 East European Ashkenazis, between 2.4 and 4.3 percent of the total population respectively (in 1800 East European Jews formed about 4.3 percent of the total East European population; see p. 27, Table 1). Both studies show that one cannot choose a model for the demographic history of Ashkenazic Jewry without some knowledge of modern demography.

Calculation of Admixture

The two articles mentioned above had a follow-up in which Xue et al. (2017) intend to provide more precise time and place of admixture that occurred among Ashkenazis in order to arrive at a model for Ashkenazic Jewish history. The article starts with a new, controversial definition of Ashkenazis, "Ashkenazic Jews [...] are individuals of Jewish ancestry with a recent origin in Eastern Europe", based on Weinryb (1973). I checked all the 29 pages on which *Ashkenaz* or derived forms are mentioned according to the index. Weinryb does not define Ashkenazis in such a way! However, Weinryb does mention German Ashkenazis (ibid., 98, 101). In view of the definition in Xue et al.'s article, East European Ashkenazis are meant.

Also in this case, the right parameters should be used to construct a historical and demographic model of Ashkenazic history. The authors mention that Ashkenazis appeared in Germany in the tenth, and in Eastern Europe in the thirteenth century. In the model of Ashkenazic history (their Figure 7), a genetic bottleneck is presented, analogous to the ones by Palamara et al. (2012) and Carmi et al. (2014) with an admixture event before and after. As shown above, these bottlenecks cannot have occurred as they result in impossible growth rates. This means that the authors must have used statistical methods and simulations that were based on wrong parameters, which makes their percentages admixture dubious. Jews lived in Eastern Europe for more than 1,000 years before the bottlenecks of Palamara and Carmi without a historical event that makes a bottleneck in Eastern Europe necessary during this period (van Straten 2017).

The conclusion that admixture first occurred in Southern Europe is in agreement with Costa et al. (2013). Xue et al. (2017) mention that South European admixture took place about 24–49 generations ago, 750–1375 CE, indicating that almost no admixture had occurred during most of the first millennium. They explain that "the group that eventually gave rise to contemporary Ashkenazis did not reside in Southern Europe until that time". The explanation does not agree with historical data. Jews were living in Italy all along the first millennium. For example, in 519 the synagogue of Ravenna was burned. Theodoric ordered the synagogue to be rebuilt (JewishEncyclopedia.com: Ravenna). In addition, 12 places in Southern Italy are mentioned up to the seventh century where Jews lived (Simonsohn 2014, 94–99). Between the fourth and the seventh century Jews were living in Sicily (Simonsohn 1997, 1–14). In 846 Nathan ben Efran died in Venosa (Jewishhistory.org.il: 846). Around 722 and 930 CE, some of the Italian Jews, from Southern Italy, arrived in the region north of the Black Sea due to anti-Jewish measures by the Byzantine emperors Leo III and Romanos I, respectively (Starr 1939, 2, 34). These Byzantine Jews are part of today's East European Ashkenazis, but the extent of their contribution is unknown (Altbauer and Taube 1992, 23; van Straten 2017).

Due to the use of wrong historical and demographic data, the percentages of admixture become dubious as well.

Ashkenazic Subpopulations

Gladstein and Hammer (2019) tried to find out "whether there are genetically distinct AJ [Ashkenazic Jewish] subpopulations [...] and if so, whether differential population growth, gene flow, or both contributed to the population differentiation". Three demographic models were tested: model 1 without differentiation between West and East European Ashkenazis; model 2 with a population split between the 2 populations and one common admixture event from Europeans; and model 3, similar to model 2 but with separate admixture events. They chose "the best model out of the three hypothesized demographic histories" with a special form of Bayesian statistics. Bayesian statistics is characterized by the use of data that were obtained earlier, the so-called priors. In this case the authors chose model 2. At this point, I should emphasize that it is crucial that the right priors are used. The authors found a genetic difference between West and East European Jews and suggested the following reason for the difference: East European Jews showed 3.6 times larger exponential growth rate than their western coreligionists, 0.25 vs. 0.069. Where did these growth rates come from? In their section *Parameter Estimates*, they write: "We fit an exponential model to the census data from the years 1170 to 1900". These data, especially the ones before 1800, are the erroneous census data by DellaPergola (2001, 22) I referred to on p. 23 that lead to growth rates of 1 percent or more that did not occur in Europe before 1800. Thus, wrong priors were used. How is it possible that they arrived at the right conclusion regarding the genetic difference between West and East European Ashkenazis using wrong priors? If wrong priors are used, no solid conclusions can be drawn, because the analysis can produce all kinds of results, including the right one. This means that even with the 1,000,000 simulations they carried out, the statistical analysis is of no use, and model 2 is thus wrong as well. Given, that East European Ashkenazis followed a different route to Eastern Europe from the route West European Jews used to Germany, this is another reason model 2 is not correct. There should be more than one admixture event, as is the case with model 3. The conclusion by Gladstein and Hammer, that the most likely model points to a differentiation between the two populations about 400 years ago, makes no sense either. It clearly refers to the Baron-Weinryb hypothesis that is outdated. Model 3 is at least a more realistic model as to the more than one admixture event. These admixture events must have taken place in different periods, starting much earlier than 400 years before the present.

Relevant German-Jewish Literature

Although this item is important for both history and genetics, I decided to add it to the chapter on genetics because of the phenomenon of blond Jews.

As mentioned in the introduction of the book, one of the most important reference works about medieval German-Jewish history is *Germania Judaica* (written in German). To the best of my knowledge, it is not referred to by geneticists who investigate the genetics of Ashkenazic Jewry. This becomes visible when they refer to the beginnings of German Jewry. As mentioned earlier, in *Germania Judaica* (Kober 1934, 71), the possibility of a continuous Jewish presence from 321 to 1423 is clearly considered a possibility. The Jewish presence was indeed continuous (Schütte and Gechter 2012). Not being familiar with *Germania Judaica* may well be the most important reason why the geneticists assume, following the Baron-Weinryb hypothesis, that East European Jews originate from Germany, as well as the impossible demographic consequences of this. Moreover, they also provide a wrong date for the beginning of German-Jewish history.

An important journal, although old, does not seem to be read by the mostly English speaking Jewish geneticists either: *Zeitschrift für Demographie und Statis-*

tik der Juden. In this journal, we find an interesting article about blond Jews (Feist 1927) that I will refer to shortly.

When discussing Jewish genetics, a phenomenon that should be mentioned is the occurrence of blond Jews. Ostrer (2012, 13) mentions the possibility that modern blond Jews are descendants of blond Israelites who lived during biblical times. His remark is based on the report that there were blond Amorites. However, the occurrence of blond Jews has not been investigated by geneticists. Considering that 18 to 30 percent of Ashkenazis are blond with blue or grey eyes – the percentage depending on the location in Europe – and that blondness is a European feature (Fishberg 1911, 78), it would be interesting to know how this phenomenon entered Ashkenazic Jewry. For example, in Germany and Austria the percentage of blond Jews is about 30 percent, in the Caucasus less than 1 percent, while in Yemen there are no fair-haired Jews at all. The admixture appears to be the most realistic explanation for the blond Jews (Fishberg 1907). The more than 80 percent of European ancestry, based on mtDNA (Costa et al. 2013), does not contradict this explanation.

In 1927, Sigmund Feist published a paper that should then have ended the notion that the Amorites and some Israelites were blond. He mentions that the blond ("*arischen*") Israelites were only invented to explain the occurrence of the blond element among today's Jews. The assumption then is that also in biblical times there were blond and blue-eyed Jews. This whole idea about blue-eyed and blond Amorites finds its origin in a mistaken observation of the Amorites on Egyptian reliefs. Feist then refers to Max Burchardt – leader of the expedition to Egypt to investigate the portrayal of foreign people – who checked the reliefs, and who wrote him the following (translated from German):

> I [...] concluded that all these blue-eyed Semites, as far as I could see the originals, rest on mistakes of the old artists! The eyes are light brown to black brown. Similarly, the hair of the Semites is never blond, but always black to dark brown, the beard as well [...] The myth of the blond Semites is related to careless observation. Many Egyptian painters put black paint on top of a yellow layer. This yellow [layer] causes the paint on top to peel off easily. And when one finds yellow blond or ash blond Semites in some grave, it means that black is not well conserved in the paintings of the whole grave! Even the Egyptians are then blond!

So much for blond Amorites and Israelites.

The fact that still today blond Jews are suggested to be descendants of blond Israelites shows again that the mostly English-speaking geneticists who are involved in Jewish genetics are not familiar with the relevant German-Jewish historiography. The German-Jewish journal may be old, but that does not mean that every article in it is outdated. Moreover, in view of Ostrer's remark mentioned in the introduction of the book, it may not be convenient to investigate the origin of the blond European Jews.

Conclusions

1. To relate genetic research to political aims is against scientific ethics; it makes manipulation appealing.
2. Mitochondrial DNA research shows contradictory results concerning the number of Ashkenazic founding mothers, due to different methodologies, and concerning the origin of Ashkenazic founding mothers, due to a combination of methodology and wrong demographic data.
3. European mtDNA lineages are the main ones in Ashkenazic Jewry.
4. The so-called ancestral Y chromosome gene pool of Ashkenazic Jewry may refer not only to Shosu and/or Apiru, but also to various kinds of Canaanite tribes as a result of intermarriage, and is thus controversial.
5. Ancient DNA of the various populations in the area of both kingdoms during biblical times may be the only way to determine who the ancestors of today's Ashkenazis (and other Jews) were.
6. Wrong demographic data cannot be used to disprove the use of uniparental markers to compare the histories of different populations, or to test the founder effect hypothesis with regards to disease alleles.
7. The biblical story about one arch-father of early Israelites and their descendants is not tenable according to archeological and genetic research.
8. Four Ashkenazic grandparents are no proof of a descent of early Israelites. They only show that the four grandparents were Ashkenazis.
9. Models based on phantom migrations cannot be used to determine the demographic history of Ashkenazic Jewry.
10. The extent of admixture cannot be determined when it is based on wrong historical and demographic data.
11. The assumption by Xue et al. that only East European Ashkenazis are Ashkenazis by descent is not right. They are only Ashkenazis by rites because they do not originate from Germany as descendants of German Jews do.
12. The articles discussed in this chapter show that even excellent genetic research misfires when it is based on wrong historical and demographic data, or when these data are used as priors.
13. German-Jewish historiography is crucial for a scientific discussion of East European Jewish history.

IV Historical and Genetic Foundations for a Southern Route

Introduction

If there is reason to believe that East European Jews originated from Judea via Anatolia and Southern Europe, instead of via Germany, there should be an indication of an early Judean/Jewish presence in these regions, and of migrations from these regions to the region around the Black Sea. In addition, a genetic difference should also be demonstrable as well if East European Jews did not originate in Germany or Bohemia. For our purpose, Anatolia may be considered as Southern Europe because, in the period under discussion, it was colonized by the Greeks.

History

The Greek Colonies and Mainland Greece

Around 1000 BCE, Greeks from mainland Greece started to migrate to the western coast of Anatolia (Rhodes 2006). The main region was Ionia, the coastal region between Miletus in the south and Phocaea in the north (see Figure 7).

Later on, from the sixth century BCE onward, they founded a number of cities around the Cimmerian Bosporus (today's Strait of Kerch) and north of the Black Sea, some of which became part of the Kingdom of the Cimmerian Bosporus (ca. 438 BCE–ca. 370 CE; see Figure 8). The Greek colonists along the Bosporus originated from Asia Minor mostly from the region between Miletus and Phocaea. The emigration was the result of the bad economic situation as a result of the wars against the Lydians that started around 768 BCE (Jeffery 1976, 211), and later on, as a result of the wars against the Persians. The only solution to solve the problems was through the emigration of part of the Ionic population (Kochelenko and Kouznetsov 1990).

The presence of Judeans in Anatolia has been recorded since the third century BCE (*Encyclopedia of Jews in the Islamic world* 2010, vol. 3, 603). For example, Miletus, Ephesus, Pergamum, and Tralles are known to have had a Judean community before and after the beginning of the Common Era (*Encyclopedia Judaica* 2007, vol. 5, 638). In Miletus is an inscription in the theatre dating from the first century BCE showing the places reserved for Judeans (Kraabel 1995, 106). Judeans lived in Ephesus from the early Hellenistic period, leading to an impor-

https://doi.org/10.1515/9783110701388-007

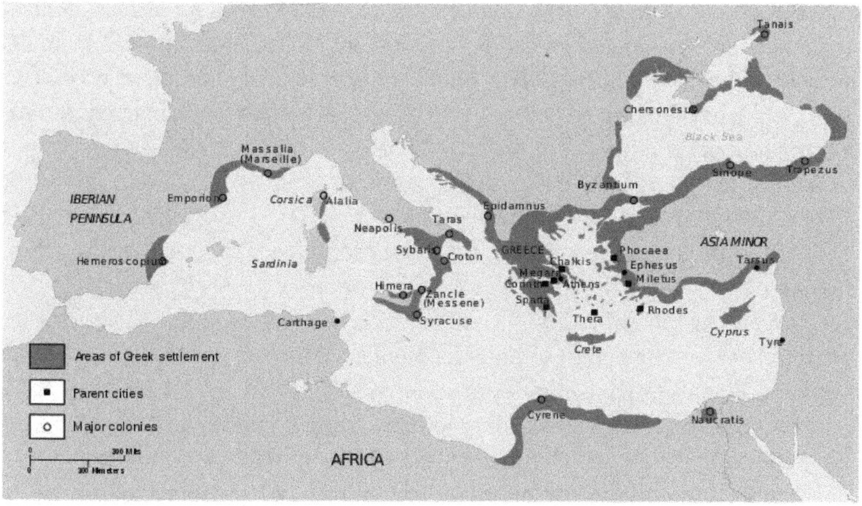

Figure 7: Greek colonies around the Mediterranean, ca. 788– ca. 500 BCE (https://en.wikipedia.org/wiki/Archaic_Greece).

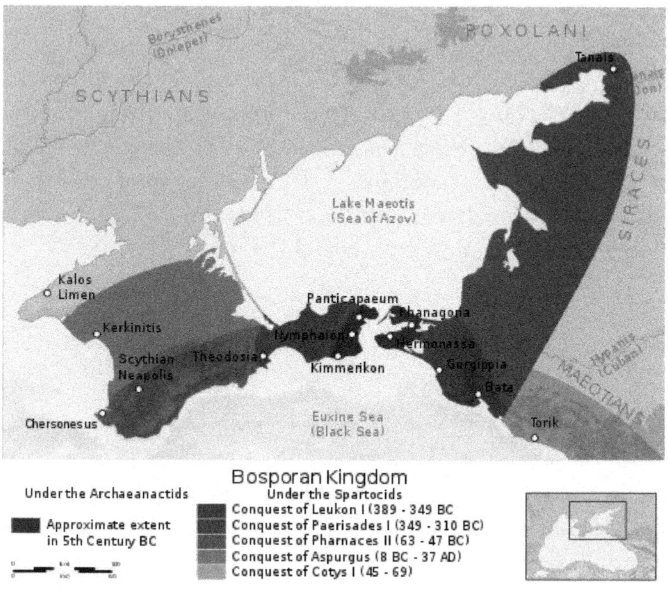

Figure 8: Kingdom of the Cimmerian Bosporus between 389 BCE and 69 CE. After 63 BCE the region was ruled by the Romans (https://en.wikipedia.org/wiki/Bosporan_Kingdom).

tant Jewish community in the first century CE, many of whom were Hellenized (*Encyclopaedia Judaica* 1930, vol. 6, Ephesos). In the sixth century CE, relatively well-to-do Jews lived in the town [ibid.]. In Smyrna, an inscription was found from around the third century CE in which a Jewish lady, named Rufina, warns the public not to bury anyone in the grave of her family under penalty of having to pay a fine to the sacred treasure, and to the Jewish nation, of 1,500 and 1,000 dinars, respectively (Reinach 1883). During this period, Jews were living in large parts of Asia Minor, for example in Ephesus, Tarsus, Armenia, and Cappadocia (ibid.).

During the time of Philo (20 BCE–50 CE), Judeans lived not only along the southern and western coast of Anatolia but also along the northwest shore in Bithynia, a Roman province that borders on Thrace (Philo, 1972, 263, [281]).

An interesting remark regarding Jewish (Judean) migrations is found in the Encyclopaedia Judaica: "Asia Minor (Anatolia) was undoubtedly also a homeland, or at least a transition station, for the Jews who established the Jewish center on the northern bank of the Black Sea" (*Encyclopaedia Judaica* 2007, vol. 5, Panticapaeum). It is therefore quite plausible that the Hellenized Judeans found in the Greek colonies around the Black Sea came from Ionia and other regions in Anatolia.

The first time a Judean is mentioned in mainland Greece is between 300 and 250 BCE in Oropos in east Attica (Lewis 1997, 380–382). At the beginning of the Common Era, Judeans lived in various parts of mainland Greece, such as Thessaly, Boeotia, Attica, Argos, and Corinth (see Figure 9), as well as Macedonia (north of Thessaly), and also on the islands of Euboea (see Figure 9), Cyprus, and Crete (Philo 1972, 263, [281], [282]). Therefore, the Judeans around the Black Sea may have come from mainland Greece and/or the islands as well.

Italy

During the same period and earlier, Judeans lived in Rome and other parts of Italy. Tacitus, who lived from ca. 56 CE to ca. 117 CE, writes that Judeans and Egyptians were expelled from Rome in 19 CE because of their religious practices. Four thousand youth (of military age) had to be shipped to Sardinia, while others had to leave Italy unless they renounced their religious practices (Tacitus 1906, no. 85). According to Stern (1980, vol. 2, 72) the number of 4,000 refers to Jews (Judeans) only, and it is an indication of the number of Jews in Rome. His conclusion is based on the singular form in Tacitus of *ea superstitione*, that superstition. The conclusion is doubtful though. If Tacitus actually only writes about the Judeans, why would he add the Egyptians? In a thorough article

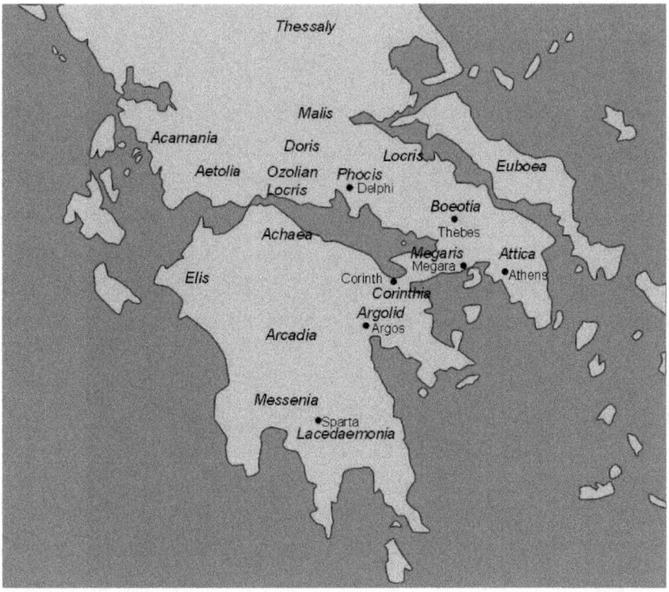

Figure 9: Various regions and towns in Greece (http://www.historyofwar.org/Maps/maps_greece_ancient_regions).

based on the number of tombs, Rutgers (2006, 354) shows that the average size of the Jewish community of Rome was 620 people at the most from the first through the fourth century CE. This size makes the number of 4000 Jewish young men unlikely as well. Furthermore, for Tacitus, who did not like the cults of either people, their religions may have been the same superstition.

Judeans and Jews around the Black Sea

Based on one manumission inscription found near Olbia (ca. last century BCE), two near Gorgippia (first century CE), and two near Kerch (one from the first century CE, one of unknown date), Harkavy (1867, 80, 4) concluded that Jews [Judeans] had lived in these towns already from before the beginning of the Common Era, that they had been completely Hellenized, and that they spoke Greek. Levinskaya (1996, 107) mentions that from the first century CE onward, there was a strong increase in the cult of *Theos Hypsistos* (θεὸς Ὕψιστος), the Highest God, in the Kingdom of the Cimmerian Bosporus. The cult became widespread by the fourth century. Furthermore, "according to the inscriptions, the worship of the Highest God was connected with Jewish synagogues from the very beginning" (ibid., 108). This is particularly clear in inscriptions that contain the word *proseuche* (προσευχή), the Greek word for synagogue. The latest inscription in this respect dates from 306 CE (ibid., 110).

Jews were present in Crimea where they joined the insurrection against the Christian bishops in Chersonesus in 300 CE (Dan'shin 1996). Up to the beginning of the fifth century, there is evidence of a Jewish presence in the Kingdom of the Cimmerian Bosporus (Levinskaya and Tokhtas'yev 1996, 5). The Greek historian Theophanes Abbas Agri et Confessor (1839, 545) writes that during the seventh century, Jews were living near Phanagoria. Israel Halpern (1960, 290) is quite clear about the Jewish presence in the region north of the Black Sea:

> If the existence of the Jewish settlement in this region during the Hellenistic period is still a matter of conjecture, there is certainty regarding the Roman period, and thereafter this region was seemingly never without a Jewish settlement.

The closeness of Greece and especially its colonies in Anatolia to the Land of Israel makes these regions likely sources for the Judeans north of the Black Sea.

Jews in Khazaria

After ca. 670, the Khazars appear on the scene, and admixture with them should not be excluded, although we have no information on this. We only know for certain that King Bulan of the Khazars converted to Judaism in 861 (Zuckerman 1995). We should realize that Jews had been living in and near the region called Khazaria for more than 850 years before King Bulan of the Khazars converted to Judaism. The following questions seem therefore justified: did his conversion add significantly more converts to the already large Jewish community? Or, was the situation maybe such that the king converted to Judaism because there were so many Jews already living in his kingdom? These questions cannot be answered as long as we do not have more information about the Khazars. And, as mentioned before, a Jew in Khazaria did not have to be a converted Khazar. Before Halpern (1960, 290) discusses the Khazars, he makes the following statement: "For more than 600 years, Jewish settlement existed only in this one corner of Eastern Europe north of the Black Sea". The long Jewish presence during the first 670 years of the Common Era may make the Khazars considerably less important for East European Jewry than assumed by some scientists (see also my comments on pp. 30 – 32).

Boulnois (1966, 189–190) writes that Qutaiba ibn Muslim expelled the Jews from Chorasmia (also named Kwarizm) south of the Aral Sea. They arrived in Khazaria,

> and included among them were numerous rabbis and scholars [...] There were already a great many Greek or ex-Syrian Jews in Khazaria, just as there were all round the Black Sea, but it seems to have been the 'secretic Judaism' of the Chorasmian Jews rather than the traditional Judaism which became the official doctrine of the Khazar State. In due course [...] Talmudic clergy were fetched from Baghdad, Khorasan and the Byzantine Empire.

However, she does not provide a reference on which this information is based.

In 721–722, the Byzantine Emperor Leo III, the Isaurian, ordered Jews to be baptized. Part of the Jews left Byzantium (Starr 1939, 2). In note 13, the author writes that around 722, "The Jews began to come [to Khazaria] from Baghdad, from Khorasan, and from the land of Greece". If Jews indeed fled to Khazaria, they must have known that it was safe for them to go there. The most logical reason for them to know that was the presence of Jews living there already. This is another indication that Jews had been living in the region for quite some time. In 873–74, Jews in Southern Italy were baptized, but nothing is known about an emigration. A second migration from Byzantium did take place though: "It is known both from this historian [al-Mas'udi] and from a Jewish source that the emperor's policy (Romanos I (919–944)) caused a considerable migration to Khazaria" (ibid., 7). Starr refers to information from ca. 930: "[...] Many Jews had migrated thither [Khazaria], having come from all the cities of the Moslems as well as from Byzantium" (ibid., 151, note 91). During this period, the Byzantine Empire included not only Greece and Anatolia but also Southern Italy and parts of the Balkans. Migrations took place from Southern Italy as well (ibid., 34):

> In the meantime, the relatively strong proportion which they [the Jews] undoubtedly constituted in Apulia, e. g., in Oria, and later in Bari and Otranto, must have diminished during the ninth and tenth centuries, primarily as a result of the emigration and destruction caused by the Moslem invasions.

But also, in this case, nothing is known about numbers.

Bartal (2017, 227) refers to the "scholars [who] have had difficulty in tracing historical continuity between the Jews who lived in the area during the Hellenistic, Byzantine, and Gothic periods and those who resided in the Slavic principalities hundreds of years later." Was there really such a discontinuity? As we saw above, Jews were living in the region in the seventh century. In the eighth and tenth centuries, Jews fled to Khazaria. Is it realistic to assume that in the

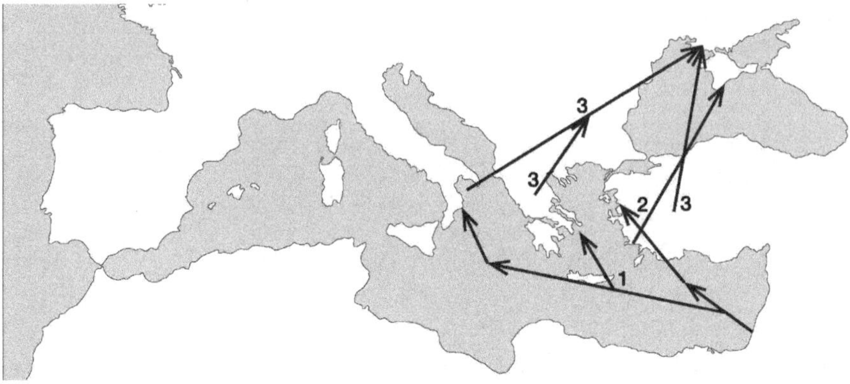

Figure 10: Major Judean/Jewish migrations leading to East European Jewry: Judean migrations from the Land of Israel to Anatolia, Greece, and Italy (1→) Judean migrations from Anatolia to the Kingdom of the Cimmerian Bosporus (2→) Jewish migrations from Byzantium (Southern Italy, Greece, Thrace, and Anatolia) to southern Ukraine (3→). The arrows in this figure indicate the beginning and endpoint only, not the routes taken (based on WHKMLA Historical Atlas http://www.zum.de/whkmla/histatlas/rome/haxromanempire.html, printed with the consent of the author, Alexander Ganse).

ninth century no Jews were living there? Were there such pogroms in those years that they all fled? Further on (ibid., 228) the author writes: "There is no doubt, for example, that between the ninth and the twelfth centuries, Jews were living in Kiev […] which had been under Khazar rule prior to the end of the tenth century."

As historical sources show that Judeans may have come to Greece (including its colonies) and Italy well before the beginning of the Common Era, followed by migrations to the area around the Black Sea (see Figure 10), the next problem to be tackled is: do genetic data agree with an origin of East European Jews via a southern route?

Genetics

The main genetic information about the maternal genetic history of Ashkenazis comes from the publication by Costa et al. (2013) who worked with mitochondrial DNA (mtDNA). As mentioned before, mtDNA is inherited from the mother. This means that we can follow the maternal line. The reason today's mtDNA can be used for following back the maternal line is that every mtDNA maintains the earlier mutations. In addition, it is possible to calculate when the earlier mutations took place. This way one can also get information about the period in which the different mutations took place.

The findings by Costa et al. have a number of points in their favor, compared to those by most other geneticists. In their article, the origin of East European Ashkenazis is not specifically tied to German Ashkenazis, as is the case for example in the article by Behar et al. (2006) who based their assumption that the major Ashkenazic mtDNA lineages originated in the Middle East partly on the assumption that Ashkenazic Jewry was "established in the 8th and 9th centuries in the Rhineland". Furthermore, Costa et al. do not use the sizes of genetic bottlenecks resulting in implausible growth rates. As we saw before, Palamara et al. (2012) and Carmi et al. (2014) found bottlenecks of some 800 Ashkenazis around 1150 and 350 Ashkenazis around 1300 respectively, resulting in implausible annual growth rates of over 1 percent (1.2 and 1.8 per cent, respectively).

Thanks to their genealogical approach, Costa et al. found that the four major founder lineages of Ashkenazic mtDNA within lineages K and N1b, namely K1a1b1a, K1a9, K2a2, and N1b2, were of European origin. These lineages had been considered as typically Jewish and were wrongly presented as an indication of a Middle Eastern origin (Behar et al. 2006). Most of the minor mtDNA Ashkenazic lineages investigated by Costa et al. originated in prehistoric Europe as well.

About 11,500 years ago, K1a1b1 arrived in Europe from the Middle East. It dates to about 11,700 years before present. K1a1b1a arose from K1a1b1 some 4400 years ago, due to three mutations. That the ages just mentioned are rather rough estimates follows from the wide range of the standard deviations, from 6800 – 16700 and from 700 – 8200 years ago for K1a1b1 and K1a1b1a, respectively (Costa et al. 2013). From 300 BCE, Judean men came to the Greek colonies in Anatolia and may have married European women carrying K1a1b1a. As a result, a mixed Judean-European community was created. The same may have happened, although somewhat later, in Rome. K1a1b1a constitutes 63 percent of the Ashkenazic K lineages and 20 percent of all Ashkenazic mitochondrial lineages. K1a9 and K2a2 account for some 36 percent of the Ashkenazic K lineages, and date to 2300 (standard deviation: 200 – 4400) and 8400 (standard deviation: 3200 – 13700) years before present, respectively (ibid.).

Another finding, one that is particularly interesting with regards to the origin of East European Ashkenazis, is the difference in lineage frequencies between West and East European Ashkenazis, for both the major and most of the minor mitochondrial lineages. As to lineage K, among West European Ashkenazis (German/Swiss) almost 50 percent of the mtDNA belongs to this lineage, while this is only 15 percent among East European Ashkenazis (in Russia) (ibid.). As long as K1a1b1a survived in Western Europe, it added to the difference in frequency between West and East European Ashkenazis via admixture. The work by Costa et al. reinforces the demographic conclusion that East European Ashkenazis do not originate from Germany.

Taking into account that East European Ashkenazis are the large majority among Ashkenazis today in the United States, England, and Israel, it is not so easy to show a difference between West and East European Ashkenazis without good genealogical research back to the last quarter of the eighteenth century.

It is plausible that, among Judeans who moved to the region around the Black Sea, there were women belonging to the Judean-European community in Greece, Italy, or Anatolia who were the source of the major and minor mtDNA lineages in East European Ashkenazis. Later, during the eighth and tenth centuries, Jewish women with their families from Byzantium (certainly Italy, and Greece) arrived in Khazaria, who may have been carriers of K1a1b1a and N1b2 (and most of the minor lineages) as well.

Founder lineages K2a2 and K1a9 also show a difference in distribution between West and East European Ashkenazis. K1a9 originated in Western Europe (ibid.). The question is: who may have brought it to Eastern Europe? This question will be discussed in the chapter on Yiddish.

There must have been more Jewish males from the Middle East than females, as it is mostly the men who went abroad as merchants or in any other capacity, but it can never have been close to 100 percent, simply from a practical point of view. It is not feasible that there was a Middle Eastern Jewish man available for every Jewish girl in Europe who wanted to get married during the centuries of a Jewish presence in Europe. And, of course, there is also genetic evidence about non-Jewish men entering the Jewish community.

Conclusions

1. Before the beginning of the Common Era, Judeans from the Greek colonies (and mainland Greece) lived in Crimea and north of it.
2. Up to the seventh century, there is documentation of a Jewish presence north of the Black Sea.
3. The early presence of Judeans and Jews north of the Black Sea makes the Khazar hypothesis implausible, as does genetic evidence.
4. During the eighth and tenth centuries, Jews from Greece and Southern Italy respectively came to Khazaria, together with Jews from Muslim places.
5. The main and almost all minor mtDNA lineages show a difference between West and East European Ashkenazis, are of European origin, and are compatible with an origin via Southern Europe and Anatolia.

V Why do East European Ashkenazis Speak Yiddish?

Introduction

Yiddish is a component language, with German as the main component. It also contains Hebrew, Slavic, and Romance words. If it is true that East European Jewry started in southern Ukraine, it does not appear logical that their descendants should speak Yiddish, a German based language. The three major hypotheses concerning the origin of Yiddish are the Rhineland hypothesis (Weinreich 1980, 329–330), the Danube hypothesis (Faber and King 1984; Katz 1985), and the Sorb hypothesis (Wexler 1991). In 2011, I suggested that a fourth hypothesis, the Bavarian-Czech hypothesis, is more appropriate to explain the origin of Yiddish in Eastern Europe. These hypotheses have also been used to explain the origin of East European Ashkenazis. I will summarize the four hypotheses and add a new argument that detaches the origin of Yiddish from the origin of East European Ashkenazis.

According to the Rhineland hypothesis, the Jews of Cologne fled to Gaul when the "barbarians", Germanic tribes, occupied the city. When, centuries later, they returned to the Rhineland, the Yiddish language had started to develop. Because nothing is known about a Jewish presence in the Rhineland between 331 and 751, but only in Gaul, Weinreich decided that they must have fled when the Germanic tribes took over the city. In addition, he shows that the name of the river Rhine, used in the Hebrew literature during the tenth century, ריינוס, transcribed as *rinus*, is a mixture of Middle High German, *rîn*, and Latin, *-us*, pointing clearly to Gaul. The use of Romance words in Cologne is no solid evidence for a return from Gaul in any case. Müller and Frings (1968, 525) write (translated from German):

> A main measure of the year 50 CE was the settlement of veterans near the colony. As a result, especially Mediterranean people entered the region [...] Following the departure of the Romans, the Roman or Romanized population may have stayed in the encampments or their surroundings for a longer period.

The idea that the Jews fled from the Rhineland when the Germanic tribes took over the city is not based on evidence. As mentioned in the introduction of the book, no group had to leave the city. This makes Weinreich's knowledge of early German history questionable. Moreover, in the 1980s, Faber and King, as well as Katz, showed, that linguistically, the Rhineland could not have been

https://doi.org/10.1515/9783110701388-008

the origin of the Yiddish language. In addition, the transcription of רינוס as *rinus* is doubtful. A more logical transcription is *renus*, the Latin name of the river. After all, Latin was one of the languages spoken in Cologne. There is every reason to assume that the Jews spoke the vernacular like they did in other countries as well.

The Danube hypothesis has become the most popular hypothesis and states that Yiddish originated in southeast Germany, where Bavarian was spoken. The idea that Yiddish originated from the Bavarian area had been suggested earlier by Mieses (1924, 269), but he did not use the name "Danube" in this respect. It appears that the German component of Yiddish is indeed derived from Bavarian.

In 1991 Wexler proposed his Sorb hypothesis: Yiddish is a Slavic language derived from Sorbian, and originated in the land of the Sorbs. Furthermore, East European Jews are mainly descendants from Sorbs, and to some extent from Khazars. Finally, Wexler is of the opinion that *ashkenaz* does not relate to Germany, but some region in ancient Persia (Das et al. 2016). Aptroot (2016) mentions in a reaction to this idea: "Wexler's theory did not gain acceptance in the scholarly community". Finally, Flegontov et al. (2016) showed that the geographic population system used by Das et al. to infer ancestry is not suitable for this purpose and that (again) Wexler's Yiddish relexification theory is unsound.

In 1998, Eggers published his Habilitationsschrift in which he proposed the Bavarian-Czech hypothesis. Salient details of this hypothesis are: the oldest Slavic words are not Sorbian but Old Czech, originally the German component was Bavarian, and religion played an important role when the language developed. Bavarian was not only spoken in Bavaria, but also in Bohemia and Moravia. The Bavarian-Czech hypothesis can be considered a modification of the Danube hypothesis. Old Czech is a logical origin for the Slavic words in Yiddish. Bohemia had famous rabbis who obviously spoke Old Czech (and Bavarian). The Old Czech origin of the glosses (Hebrew words translated into Old Czech, also called West Slavic Canaanite) in rabbinical medieval Hebrew manuscripts, also in Germany and France, was recently proven by Dittmann (2017, 234–283). There were students speaking Old Czech (or Old Polish that was very similar) who visited the Talmud schools in France and Germany. For these students, the Slavic words were probably included in Hebrew commentaries of the Torah and Talmud. It goes without saying that rabbis in Bohemia used Old Czech words in their Hebrew commentaries as well.

The most plausible assumption is that Yiddish indeed originated from Bohemia (and Moravia) where the rabbis spoke Bavarian, Old Czech, and knew Hebrew.

A linguistic phenomenon known as unrounding of vowels (*ü* becomes *i* and *ö* becomes *e*), found in all Yiddish dialects, first occurred around 1200 in parts of

Bohemia and Moravia (Eggers 1998, 227). This is an important observation because it means that Yiddish did not originate before ca. 1200.

There were possibly family relationships between the Bohemian/Moravian and German or French rabbis. Zunz (1859, 73) reports that the twelfth-century Bohemian rabbis Isaac halaban ben Jacob, Eliezer ben Isaac, and Isaac ben Mordekhai lived in Germany as well. Daughters of rabbis normally married sons of rabbis. The Romance words in Yiddish may have come from contacts between the rabbis from Bohemia and Moravia and rabbis from France and Germany.

With a low level of religious knowledge among East European Ashkenazis before 1200, the obvious persons to teach East European Ashkenazis Yiddish would be rabbis and teachers of religion who spoke Yiddish (Zinberg 1975, 6). In the beginning, these people must have come from Germany or Bohemia and Moravia where the level of Jewish knowledge was very high. It was found that founder lineage K1a9 originated in the West. It amounts only to 6 percent of all main Ashkenazic lineages in Eastern Europe (Costa et al. 2013). One such source could be some of the women of the aforementioned rabbis and/or teachers. Women of rabbis from Bohemia and Moravia who went to Eastern Europe may have been a source as well. This means that K1a9 occurred initially in a limited group. It would also explain why, later on, K1a9 occurred in Eastern Europe at a much lower frequency than K1a1b1a. One could explain the differences in frequencies by genetic drift. However, the authors tried to diminish this possibility by using the diversity and the nesting structure in the tree for most of the inferences.

Jews Spoke the Vernacular

As mentioned above, before and shortly after the beginning of the Common Era, Judeans around the Black Sea must have spoken Greek. Later on, their descendants must have switched to a Slavic language, because a Slavic language became the vernacular, and the Jews, as everywhere else in those days, spoke the vernacular. Do we have evidence that East European Ashkenazis indeed spoke a Slavic language before they spoke Yiddish? The Jews who lived in Eastern Europe before 1200 must have spoken the vernacular because the Yiddish language uses unrounded vowels, and as we saw before, unrounding only started around that time. The arguments I put forward earlier (van Straten 2011a, 126–127), for example how at the beginning of the seventeenth century rabbis mentioned in *responsa*, that most of the Jews spoke Russian, and that in 1650 there were still regions in Russia where the Jews only spoke Russian, confirm this view. I would like to add a few more arguments.

There is indirect information that East European Ashkenazis first spoke a Slavic language. In his book *Kitâb al-masâlik wa'l-mamâlik* (*The book of the roads and the kingdoms*), Ibn Khordadbih (c. 825–ca. 912) tells us about Jewish merchants, Radhanites, who traveled from Western Europe to China and back (de Goeje 1889, 114–115). They spoke Arabic, Persian, Romance languages, the Frankish language, Andalusian, and a Slavic language. It is not plausible that every merchant traveled the whole route: "few if any of the caravans ever traveled the whole way, some nine thousand miles there and back. Chinese merchants were never seen in Rome, nor were Roman traders in Ch'ang-an" (Hopkirk 1980, 21–22). It is also not likely that every Radhanite spoke all these languages. We may, therefore, assume that the Slavic-speaking Jewish merchants lived in a Slavic-speaking country. This would not disagree with the finding that the East Asian mitochondrial lineage M33c, most likely Chinese, was found only among East European Ashkenazis, whose ancestors couldn't have spoken Yiddish during this early period (Tian et al. 2015). But there is direct evidence as well.

In his analysis of the Jewish translation of the Vilnius Codex 262 into Belarusian, Altbauer and Taube (1992, 23) write:

> We do know, however, that the Jewish population in the area [Lithuania] included 'autochthonous' Jews who had originally migrated to Eastern Europe from the Byzantine periphery. Antedating the great immigration of Yiddish-speaking Jews from Ashkenaz [...] they spoke later Slavic [...] The process of their 'Ashkenazization' took many generations [...] the authors of the translations [...] were indeed Jewish, descendants of the 'autochthonous' Jews described above [...].

Moshe Taube of the Hebrew University in Jerusalem wrote the following: "Now, of course, there were Jews in Eastern Europe before the arrival of the Ashkenazis, and of course, like in every other diaspora, they spoke the local language. This is uncontroversial" (personal communication). Aslanov (2010, 312ff) uses the Hebrew name *kena'anim* for these Jews.

A difference between Lithuanian Yiddish and the rest of East European Yiddish is the switch that occurred long ago whereby the phoneme [ʃ] became an [s] (*shin* (*sh*) was pronounced as *samekh* (*s*)). For example, *shabbos* is pronounced *sabbos*. Aslanov investigated this phenomenon and concluded that before the *kena'anim* arrived in Lithuania, they spoke Belarusian. The switch was an adaptation to the vernacular of the region where they arrived in Lithuania.

The fact that East European Jews spoke the vernacular of the Slavic country in which they lived before they spoke Yiddish may be part of the reasons that they developed different dialects of Yiddish. Certainly, the loan words refer to the specific regions. These dialects are Lithuanian Yiddish, spoken in roughly

Lithuania, Belarus, and Latvia; Polish Yiddish, spoken in Poland and western Galicia; and Ukrainian Yiddish, spoken in Volhynia and Podolia.

The Language-cum-ethnic Shift

In Eastern Europe, we are dealing with a linguistic replacement. An appropriate model for the replacement of Slavic by Yiddish is provided by the "language-cum-ethnic shift" (Ehret 1988). The Jews in Eastern Europe were mostly living in villages and small towns (*shtetls*):

> Communities of those eras adopted objects and practices through direct encounter with people of other communities because of their practical value or because they admired or desired the traits or looked up to the people from whom the traits came, or for both reasons conjoined (ibid.).

The people to whom East European Jews looked up were the rabbis who came from the west. As mentioned before, the level of religious knowledge was very low among East European Jews. The trait in question was the *nusah ashkenaz*, the German Jewish rites the rabbis brought along. The rabbis spoke Yiddish. Although Ehret speaks of an encounter of whole community to whole community, the influence of the rabbis was probably strong enough to warrant the following:

> the embedding of the admired features of culture in the wider cultural matrix of the donor society [in this case the rabbis] could trigger off the adoption of additional parts of that matrix, undermining the sense of ethnic distinctiveness among the adopting community and leading over a period of several generations to their adoption of the language and assumption of the self-identification of the donor community [the rabbis] (ibid.).

The language-cum-ethnic shift fits the situation in Eastern Europe perfectly. It would also explain why East European Jewish history scholars and linguists maintain that East European Jewry originates from Germany, and why they deny that they are to some extent descendants of the Jews who lived around the Black Sea at the beginning of the Common Era. Stampfer (2012, 128) maintains that the latter did not survive the Mongol invasion. As Menache (1996) indicates, the Mongols treated the Jews the same way as non-Jews. There is no evidence to believe that Stampfer is right.

The question remains, however, of how women learned to speak Yiddish. It is known that today's women of ultra-orthodox Jews (Hebrew: *haredim*) are taught Jewish law by other women. It is plausible that when rabbis started to go to Eastern Europe and encountered a more or less ignorant Jewish community, the women were taught Jewish law by, for example, the wives of the rabbis. Laws pertaining to menstruation (Hebrew: *nida*) and kosher food (Hebrew: *kashrut*) were especially important and had to be taught. Through such contacts, women became acquainted with Yiddish as well.

It is thus possible to explain that East European Ashkenazis spoke Yiddish in the end, with only a small number of them originating from a German-speaking area. As we will see in the next chapter, a similar development must have taken place in Turkey where Jews switched from the vernacular to Judeo-Spanish. In addition to historical and genetic arguments, we now also have linguistic arguments to support a southern route for the development of East European Ashkenazis.

As to the Turkish Jews, a common comment is: "In Turkey, the Spanish speakers were more numerous than the locals and thus their culture and language dominated most communities." This idea seems to be widespread. Although Sephardic Jews are not the topic of this book, I will deal with this comment in the next chapter.

Conclusions

1. Judeans/Jews living in the Greek colonies in Anatolia or around Crimea before and after the beginning of the Common Era spoke the vernacular, i.e. Greek.
2. In time, the vernacular became a Slavic language.
3. The switch from a Slavic language to Yiddish is explained according to Ehret's language-cum-ethnic shift model.
4. Yiddish speaking women (wives of rabbis) who taught religious laws to East European Jewish women taught them Yiddish as well.

VI Are Turkish Jews Sephardic Jews?

Introduction

Sephardic Jews are Jews who lived in Iberia during the Middle Ages, and their descendants. The latter went mainly to France, England, the Netherlands, Germany, Italy, Anatolia (Turkey), North Africa, and the Americas. It is unknown how many Jews went to each country.

In 2003, Behar et al. wrote that "current usage applies this [Sephardic] designation to all descendants of the communities of North Africa and the Near East who follow the Sephardic rite of worship and cultural traditions." More specifically, in 2008, Behar et al. concluded that Turkish Jews are to be considered as Sephardic Jews. This chapter is based on a reaction to this conclusion that I placed in *PloS One* in September 2017, the journal in which the article by Behar et al. was published. It shows that controversial results in the genetic literature are not limited to Ashkenazis only.

The conclusion by Behar et al. (2008) that Turkish Jews are representatives of Iberian Jewry is mainly based on three pieces of information: statements by the interviewees; the Turkish Jews only settled in the country after the expulsion from Iberia in 1492; and Turkish Jews had mtDNA lineage HV0 that was also found among Portuguese Jews in Belmonte. I will take a closer look at these three points. In addition, the following will be discussed: the rise of the domination of Sephardic Jewry, Judeo-Spanish, and the number of Iberian surnames.

Statements by the Interviewees

The interviewees had declared that their ancestors had arrived from Spain. Genetic research by Need et al. (2009) pertaining to Ashkenazis in the United States showed that the origin of more than 45 percent of the grandparents of the Jewish interviewees was unknown: a place the grandparents left about 100 to 150 years earlier. Here, we are dealing with ancestors who supposedly left Iberia some 500 years ago. How reliable is the information about Iberia, and how can it be verified? Moreover, information about origin may be incorrect as will be explained under the heading Judeo-Spanish.

https://doi.org/10.1515/9783110701388-009

Turkish Jews only Settled in the Country after 1492

The early presence of Jews in Turkey, and especially in Anatolia, has been mentioned already on p. 62. There is a map with some 13 Jewish settlements in Turkey during the twelfth and thirteenth centuries, in addition to the one in Constantinople (Bowman 1985, 51). In 1324 Jews were living in Bursa (Encyclopedia of Jews in the Islamic world. 2010, vol. 3, 603), while in 1365 there were Jews in Edirne, which also had the first Ashkenazic community (ibid., 604). Already before the conquest of Constantinople in 1453 the city had Romaniot, Ashkenazic, Italian, and Karaite communities (Rozanes 1908, 25). Romaniots (Ῥωμανιῶτες) are neither Sephardic nor Ashkenazic Jews. They have been living in Greece, in western Asia Minor, and on the Balkans (Lewis 1987, 120) for a long time. As mentioned earlier, the first time a Jew was mentioned in Greece, was around 250 BCE. They spoke Greek.

Karaites only recognize the laws of the Old Testament, contrary to the mainstream of Jews who follow the Old Testament, the Talmud, and other rabbinical laws.

Heyd (1953) enumerates the different Jewish congregations in Istanbul in the seventeenth century. They are divided into two groups, those whose ancestors were forced to move to Istanbul by Mehmed II after he conquered Istanbul in 1453 and those who came of their own accord. The former, 22 congregations (one consisting of Karaites from Edirne), all came from within the Ottoman Empire. Ten came from Turkey itself, 8 from Greece, 3 from what is called today the Republic of North Macedonia, and 1 from Bulgaria. They must have been mainly Romaniots. The action by Mehmed II shows that Jewish communities existed in Turkey in the fifteenth century well before 1453. In the second group, we find congregations including: Portugal, Catalonia, Hamon (Granada), Ashkenazis (Germany), *Gerush* (Hebrew for expulsion, probably from Spain), Great Sicilian, Little Sicilian, Shalom Aragon, Cordova, Calabria, Cana (Salonika), and Messina. The Jewish community of Constantinople consisted clearly of Jews from various regions within Turkey and Europe, including Iberia.

Numerical Information about the Different Jewish Groups

When Behar et al. consider the entire Turkish-Jewish community as Sephardic Jews, they should first have investigated how many Jews arrived from Iberia in relation to the Jews already present. They mention "the migration of a considerable fraction of Iberian Jewish exiles to Anatolia", which is neither based on numerical data nor does it provide a numerical clue. According to Inalcik (1970,

207), Mehmed II successfully tried to settle European Jews in Constantinople. As a result, in 1477, there were 1,647 European Jewish families. In Istanbul alone, in 1478 there were more than 8,200 Romaniot and Karaite Jews (Encyclopedia of Jews of the Islamic world 2010, vol. 3, 604).

Levy (1994, 126, note 25) provides a very good discussion about the problems related to the value of numerical information about the period under discussion. In addition to the fact that the Jews did not want to be counted because the data were used by the Turkish authorities for tax purposes, there is a major problem with the interpretation of the Turkish term for household used in the registers. The number of people in a household may have varied from a husband and his family to several families. Levy continues:

> it is important to note that the information contained in the Ottoman registers has the advantage of being grounded in reality. It is, therefore, superior by far to any other sources, such as travelers' accounts, whose numbers are generally based on hearsay. Although fragmentary and deficient, the Ottoman records allow us, nevertheless, to form an approximate idea, within certain parameters, of the population size; they give us a sense of the relative strength of each group in a given location and its relative economic position; and they allow us to follow long-range demographic and economic trends.

He provides the following information based on Heyd (1953) and Epstein (1980, 186–188) (ibid., 8):

> Around the turn of the seventeenth century, the total number of recorded Jewish households in Istanbul, "old" and "new," was 2,195. Of these, Romaniot Jews still comprised more than half, whereas the immigrant congregations amounted to only about 44 percent of the households. This suggests that Jewish immigration to Istanbul, while considerable, was not on as large a scale as generally believed [...] Thus [...] the Sephardic congregations accounted for less than 25 percent of all the recorded Jewish households in Istanbul; and even if we were to include the two unidentified groups with the Sephardim, their combined numbers of 628 households would constitute less than 29 percent of the Jewish households.

The old congregations consisted of Romaniots, Ashkenazis, and, Karaites. The new ones were Sephardic, Italian, Ashkenazic, Hungarian, and two unidentified Jews. It should be mentioned here that the Italian Jews did not consider themselves as Ashkenazic or Sephardic Jews. Interesting in this respect is what happened during the middle of the eighteenth century, when a substantial number of poor Jews from Italy and some from Morocco came to Amsterdam, and declared that they were Iberian Jews. The economic situation in Amsterdam was not very good. Many poor Jews were dependent on poor relief by the Portuguese Jewish community. With a substantial number of new Jews from Italy and Morocco, the amount of money of the Portuguese community for the poor threatened to become insufficient. The leaders of the Portuguese community demanded evidence of an Iberian origin from their old communities (Rodrigues Pereira and Snel 2019). This measure clearly concerned Jews without typical Iberian surnames. The suspicion was that poor Italian or Moroccan Jews would come to Amsterdam to make use of the relief money of the Portuguese community.

Genetics

The HV0 lineage is mentioned by the authors as an indication of Iberian origin, because Jews from Belmonte, Portugal had this haplotype. However, HV0 is one of the most common lineages in the Republic of North Macedonia, which also belonged to the Turkish Ottoman Empire. Nogueiro et al. (2014) found that the presence of HV0 is not a general feature of the Sephardic Jews in Portugal. Thus, it is questionable if this lineage is evidence of an Iberian Jewish origin. The data in the above section also cast a different light on the conclusion by Behar et al. that the high variation they found reflects high overall mtDNA diversity among Jews of Spanish descent. A more plausible explanation is that the diversity is due to the heterogeneity of the Turkish Jewish community. Meanwhile, the idea that Turkish Jews are Sephardic was adopted by other geneticists who investigated the genetics of Sephardic Jews (Adams et al. 2008; Atzmon et al. 2010). Trombetta et al. (2015) investigated Sephardic-Turkish Jews with regards to sub-lineages E-M34 and E-M81 (Table 4).

The DNA of the Turkish Jews in Table 4 was labeled by the National Laboratory for the Genetics of Israeli Populations as Sephardic Jews from Turkey. It is questionable if the laboratory did extensive genealogical research about these “Sephardic” Jews. The data show that, in addition to the heterogeneity of the Turkish Jews, they probably intermarried with Turkish non-Jews as well. Although E-M81 was also present in Portuguese and Spanish non-Jews, it is more likely that admixture took place with Turks because of the good relations between Jews and Turks in the Ottoman Empire. If E-M34 and E-M81 would have been lineages that occurred among Jewish Judeans, it is strange that we do not find these lineages among Ashkenazis. It is not plausible that Jews with E-M34 and E-M81 would have gone only to Iberia. Although E-M81 occurred in the Portuguese and Spanish individuals sampled as well – varying from 2.2 to 41.1 percent – E-M34 was only found among one Iberian group, Asturians, with only 1.1 percent. Both E-M81 and E-M34 were also found among southwestern Turks, northeastern Turks, and Turkish Cypriots. These data indicate that these Sephardic-Turkish Jews are, in addition to being a mixture of Ashkenazic, Sephardic,

Italian, and Romaniot Jews, also partly Turkish, and should not be considered Sephardic.

Table 4: Frequencies (%) of E-M34 and E-M81, sub-lineages of E-M215 among Sephardic and non-Jewish Turks, Continental Greeks, Sephardic Bulgarians and Italians (from Trombetta et al. (2015), Table S7).

	Frequencies of sub–lineages of E-M215 %	
Population	E-M34	E-M81
Sephardic Turkish	5.3	5.3
Istanbul Turkish	2.9	5.7
Southwestern Turkish	2.5	2.5
Northeastern Turkish	0,0	2.4
Central Anatolian	3.3	0.0
Southeastern Turkish	4.2	0.0
Ezurum Turkish	8.0	0.0
Turkish Cypriots	2.2	8.7
Continental Greeks	3.1	0.0
Sephardic Bulgarians	5.0	0.0
Italy (average)	3.6	0.9

Domination of Sephardic Jewry

Well into 1600, the Romaniots were the dominant group in Istanbul, not the Sephardic Jews (Levy 1994, 61). From then on Sephardic influence increases, both economically and religiously. Although the other Jewish congregations tried to maintain their own identity, this was not possible in the end. Some of the first to adopt the Sephardic culture, including their language, were the Italian congregations (Heyd 1953). The Ashkenazis followed suit. The two communities that were most resistant to Sephardic influence were the Karaites and the Romaniots, the oldest Jewish communities in the country (ibid.). The Romaniots had been the largest Jewish congregation until well into the seventeenth century (Levy 1994, 8). Nevertheless, after 1600, the Romaniot community began to mix with the Sephardic community and eventually became part of it leading up to the Sephardic Turkish community.

Judeo-Spanish and Iberian Surnames

The fact that Turkish Jews speak Judeo-Spanish has been interpreted as evidence that Turkish Jews originate from Iberia. However, as is the case with Yiddish (see p. 75), we are dealing here also with linguistic replacement, according to Ehret's "ethnic-cum-language shift" model (Ehret, 1988). Again, a relatively small foreign group of Jews, this time from Iberia, with a higher educational and cultural level – at the most 29 percent of the Jewish population in Istanbul at the beginning of 1600 – entered an extensive region with Jews of lower religious knowledge. As mentioned above, the local Jewish populations adopted the customs of the immigrants, some rather quickly, some, following a tough opposition to the Iberians, at a later stage. In the end, most Turkish Jews spoke Judeo-Spanish and had the idea – as is shown by the interviewees – that they originated from Iberia as well, similar to the East European Ashkenazis who think that they originate from Germany.

If the Turkish Jews would indeed be descendants of Iberian Jews, we should find that most of the surnames of the Turkish Jews are Iberian the way we find Iberian surnames in Amsterdam or Hamburg among the Portuguese/Spanish Jews. In a list with 99 Jewish surnames of Turkey (http://www.angelfire.com/wy/yaw/jewish.html) taken down by Daniel Kazez from Yusuf Betsalel's book *Osmanli ve Turk Yahudileri*, only 14 were Spanish.

The above mentioned historical, genetic, and demographic data show that Turkish Jews cannot be considered a genetic continuation of Sephardic Jewry. Turkish Jews are a mixture of Romaniot, Italian Ashkenazic, and Sephardic Jews, and Turks. At the beginning of the seventeenth century, Sephardic Jews were still a minority among the Turkish Jews, and it is quite feasible that they still are. This heterogeneity also explains the high overall mtDNA diversity among the Turkish Jews and the relatively small number of Iberian surnames.

The question remains of why a geneticist would consider Turkish Jews as Sephardic Jews when there is so much historical evidence that they are a mixture of Romaniots, Ashkenazic and Italian Jews, and Turks. It reminds me of some Dutch Ashkenazis, referred to on p. 46, who maintain that they are Sephardic Jews

Conclusions

1. Jews lived in Turkey from the third century BCE.
2. At the beginning of the seventeenth century, the majority of Turkish Jews still consisted of Romaniots.

3. Turkish Jews are a mixture of Ashkenazic, Sephardic, Italian, and Romaniot Jews, and are also partly Turkish.
4. Because of the high cultural level of the Sephardic immigrants, Judea-Spanish became the vernacular of the Turkish Jews according to Ehret's "ethnic-cum-language shift" model.

Summary

In view of the involvement of different disciplines in this study before and after the beginning of the Common Era, it may be helpful to summarize the main conclusions.

1. It is unknown where the early Israelites came from, and how they were interrelated. Archaeological finds indicate that the Israelites were certainly not descendants of an arch-father who lived about 3500 years ago (see also point 12).
2. It is unknown to what extent Israelites intermarried with the non-Israelites in their heterogeneous surroundings.
3. From both foregoing points, it is clear that, as long as we do not have ancient DNA of the Israelites, we do not know to whom DNA lineages of modern Jews refer to.
4. It is not possible to consider Israelites (or Judeans) direct ancestors of modern Jews because the former used a patrilineal system (the father determines the status) and the latter use a matrilineal system (the mother determines the status) including a quantitatively unknown inflow of converts, as indicated by the geographically determined Jewish phenotypes.
5. There are Ashkenazis by descent, originally from Germany, and Ashkenazis according to religious rites.
6. It is not possible to use the West model life tables of Coale and Demeny to defend invented and implausible high Jewish growth rates in Eastern Europe between 1500 and 1800.
7. Migration of Jews from the Czech lands, Silesia, and the former German eastern territories during the period after 1550 does not solve the problem of the implausible East European Jewish population increases.
8. The possibility that East European Ashkenazis are mainly descendants of Khazars is strongly reduced by the fact that the ancestors of the Ashkenazis had already lived in the relevant region already for more than 650 years before the Khazars appeared in the region, and more than 850 years before King Bulan converted to Judaism.
9. The genetic evidence for a Khazar ancestry by Elhaik is inaccurate both demographically and genetically.
10. Most of the DNA research pertaining to lay-Jews is based on incorrect historical and demographic data (Baron-Weinryb hypothesis), and leads to incorrect conclusions.

https://doi.org/10.1515/9783110701388-010

11. Via a genealogical approach, it was shown that the mtDNA profile of West and East European Ashkenazis showed a genetic difference between the two groups.
12. Determination of the Jewish Y-chromosomal ancestral gene pool led to five different lineages, which implies that the ancestors were not descendants of an arch-father who lived about 3500 years ago (see also point 1)
13. Genetic research pertaining to Jewish priests shows different lineages that also make it impossible that Aaron (brother of Moses) was the forefather of the Jewish priests. A similar problem pertains to Levites.
14. The fact that King Jeroboam I appointed Jewish priests from the "elite" of the country further justifies the former point, and also makes it unclear who the ancestors of today's priests are.
15. It is possible that the quantitative relations between the different Y-chromosomal lineages of today's Ashkenazic priests, are different from those of the Judean priests. The reason for the differences is that for the former, these differences depend on, for example, the number of priests that came to Europe with a certain lineage. The same holds for the Levites.
16. The conclusion that Yeshaya Horowitz, forefather of the rabbinic Horowitz family, originates from Spain is based on amateurish genealogical research, and is incorrect.
17. The conclusion that four Jewish grandparents are proof of a Middle Eastern origin is based on a lack of historical knowledge, and as we saw in points 1 and 2, a Middle Eastern origin does not necessarily mean an Israelite or Judean origin.
18. Studies with autosomal DNA that use demographic models with wrong parameters lead to wrong conclusions.
19. The use of Bayesian statistics to choose the right demographic model for showing substructure among Ashkenazis does not lead to usable conclusions because the chosen model is based on wrong priors.
20. The idea that there were blond Amorites and Israelites is based on wrong observations.
21. Knowledge of the German-Jewish literature about the Middle Ages is essential for a good understanding of the origin of East European Jewry.
22. The presence of Judeans from Anatolia and Greece in the Greek colonies around Crimea from before the beginning of the Common Era has been historically proven. These Judeans formed part of the ancestors of East European Jewry.
23. An origin of East European Ashkenazis via the southern route is also defendable from a genetic point of view.

24. The switch of a Slavic-speaking Jewish population to Yiddish can be explained by Ehret's language-cum-ethnic shift model.
25. From the foregoing 24 conclusions, it follows that there are two kinds of Ashkenazis, by descent and by religious rites, who differ also genetically. In both populations, the women are mainly of European origin. It is not clear if the men are descendants of the biblical Israelites, because the genetic makeup of the latter is unknown.
26. Historical, demographic, and genetic data show that Turkish Jews are not a continuation of Sephardic Jewry.
27. At the beginning of the seventeenth century, Sephardic Jews were still a minority among the Turkish Jews. At that time, the Romaniots were still the largest congregation.
28. The use of Judeo-Spanish by Turkish Jews can also be explained by Ehret's language-cum-ethnic shift model.

Epilogue

An epilogue is the place where an author has the opportunity to give his or her thoughts free reign. There are a number of matters related to the origin of some of the ethnic Jewish groups that I find troublesome from a scientific or moral point of view. I hope that the reader does not take offense at my open-heartedness about the biased way Jewish medieval history and genetics are often treated in the scientific community.

As to history, it may be helpful to start with the beginning of German-Jewish history. I am appalled at the way modern historians deal with early German-Jewish history. When did Jews arrive in Germany? Most of today's Jewish historians acknowledge a Jewish presence in Cologne in the fourth century, but deny a continuous presence between that period and the eighth or ninth century when the Jews supposedly returned to Germany. According to *Germania Judaica*, the German-Jewish reference work on medieval Jewish history in the German-speaking realm, they arrived sometime before the fourth century in Cologne. Although there is no evidence in historical sources of a Jewish presence in Cologne or somewhere else in Germany between 330 and the ninth century, *Germania Judaica* doesn't rule out the possibility that Cologne was inhabited by Jews continuously during that period. Recent archaeological work by Sven Schütte showed that the synagogue that had been assumed to be of the eleventh century, in reality, was Carolingian (eighth to ninth centuries), with an uninterrupted architectural continuity in several phases back to the fourth century and that there was, beyond serious doubts, a continuous Jewish presence from the fourth century on. Although, at first received with enthusiasm, even rabbis from Israel came to visit the archaeological site, some Jewish historians began to disagree with Schütte's findings. I attended a symposium on the archaeological finds in Cologne in 2012. I was shocked by the vehement way Schütte was attacked by German archaeologists, even about his Carolingian synagogue (what Doppelfeld in 1958 had already suggested). Not only that, these days there is even a tendency to deny the presence of a Jewish community in Cologne in the Late Antiquity altogether. It is a riddle to me what is going on with the discussion about an early Jewish presence in Cologne. The situation escalated, and Cologne/German politicians started to get involved. It is unclear who turned to the politicians, but in the end Schütte was dismissed, the project was "reduced" by two thirds, many houses and parts of the synagogue were destroyed, and the excavation was continued with machines (instead of by hand – the way archaeology should be carried out). As a result, much of the evidence was destroyed, especially 90 percent of the evidence of the early period. What were the underlying reasons that led to

https://doi.org/10.1515/9783110701388-011

the partial destruction of the dig? Of course, Schütte's conclusions about a continuous Jewish presence are in disagreement with East European Jewish assumptions that the beginnings of a Jewish presence in Germany was only around the ninth century, but still. Unthinkable.

In the introduction of the book, I mentioned the statement by Harry Ostrer about genetic research of Jews. It seems that his statement is merely a confirmation of a practice that had started earlier, namely trying to prevent the publication of results that do not agree with generally accepted traditional ideas about Jews, or with an origin from the Middle East. I already referred to the silencing to death of Zoossmann-Diskin's article in 2000 in the English genetic literature that showed that the Cohen modal haplotype is no Jewish lineage at all. This was not an isolated case.

It is sad that the field of Jewish genetics has become the subject of political ideas. What makes things worse is that these ideas are based on wrong assumptions. According to Ostrer, there is a straight relationship between origin (or historical rights) and territory. Before going into his statement, I would like to give an example of origin and territory in nature. If I may consider my cat as being part of nature, he has a territory of some 2400 square meters, our property. It is not his territory because his mother, grandfather, or any other relative came from here, but because he can defend it. As to humans, it is unbelievable that an American scientist would come up with such a statement. If there is one good example of a country that clearly shows that such a relationship does not exist, it is the United States. For all practical purposes, the United States is run by "Europeans". The Native Americans who have been living there for more than 15,000 years, and did not leave, have nothing to say as far as ruling the country is concerned. They were placed in reservations. Historical rights? The United States is not unique in this respect, with Australia and New Zealand good examples as well. I am not accusing these countries; I am merely observing how human nature and history work.

In 1948 Jewish politicians used the idea of historical rights to obtain more support for the establishment of a Jewish state. Maybe they believed that this relationship indeed exists, or maybe they just used it to reach their goal. However, there is no straightforward relationship between origin and territory in nature outside *Homo sapiens* and, as shown above, also not among *Homo sapiens*. Only one thing is important: the power to defend a territory. This may not sound very nice, but it is the reality. Do politicians and geneticists realize that the link between origin/historical rights and territory is not only an illusion, but that it exists apparently for Israel only? It seems that even historians do not realize that this link does not exist. In an earlier publication (van Straten 2011a, 199–201) I discussed the view by Sand (2010) who maintains that the

Jews had no right to the Land of Israel because they did not descend from the Israelites. Besides the fact that this link does not exist, Sand is politically motivated which means that his view becomes *a priori* questionable. But even a well-known historian like Toch does not seem to realize that the link does not exist. In his rebuttal of Sand's view (2013, 155), he only mentions that such a view is "far-fetched". It does not make any difference whether an article concludes that today's Jews do or do not originate from the Middle East. The origin argument against the State of Israel is simply not a correct argument. I never heard the argument about the origin of the non-native Americans who are ruling the United States being used against their legitimacy to rule the country. More importantly, when the "historical rights" argument is left out of the discussion, an objective discussion about the origin of today's Jews could take place. Such a discussion would not be in contradiction with the rabbinical definition of Jews that does not take origin into account anyway.

Another issue that bothered me was the assumption that specifically colored Jews are descendants of converts. This might well be due to the fact that our ideas about the origin of Ashkenazic Jewry have been developed within Europe by historians who considered the European phenotype of European Jews as the "normal" Jewish type. In other words, white European Jews are straight descendants of Judeans and Israelites. When I visited Israel in 1958, I was amazed to see Indian tourists because, in those days, Israel didn't have a friendly relationship with India yet. My amazement increased, even more, when I found out that these "tourists" were Indian Jews. They were the first colored Jews I had ever met. They didn't look "Jewish". But what did they think when they saw me? I probably didn't look Jewish to them either, despite my dark brown hair and beard (at least in those days). Is there such a thing as to look "Jewish"? When we look at the definition of a "Jew", the bit about conversion in combination with the different phenotypes among Jews makes it impossible to say that someone looks Jewish. My own experience in this matter is rather amusing. While studying in the United States, I met American Jews whom I told that I was Jewish. The response I sometimes received was: "you are Jewish, with a name like van Straten?". If my surname had been Goldstein, I probably wouldn't have had to tell them that I was Jewish; I would have looked typically Jewish. Many East European (Galician) Jews probably don't know that their German surnames are the result of a decree by the Empress Maria Theresa around 1772 that Jews had to use German names.

Ashkenazic Jewry, and especially East European Jewry, has become the dominant group of Jews after World War II. Almost all of today's Jewish scientists who are involved in Jewish history and genetics are from Eastern Europe. Most Jewish geneticists who investigate the origin of Ashkenazic Jewry follow the

Baron-Weinryb hypothesis (see p. 5), and consider Ashkenazis as Jews who genetically resemble Judeans and Israelites more than the other groups do. The Sephardic Jews may be an exception, but not the way these geneticists try to define also Bulgarian, Moroccan, and Turkish Jews as Sephardic.

The amazing part of the conclusions concerning Ashkenazis is that the geneticists involved do not seem to realize that Ashkenazis look as European – and not only the blond ones – as Indian Jews look like Indians, or as many Moroccan Jews look like Berbers. How do we know that Judeans and Israelites, who themselves were mixtures of other peoples, looked like we do? I can imagine that inhabitants of the Middle East did not look like Chinese or San people. But is that a reason to assume that they were whites? What about some kind of an "in-between type"? For example, the Yemenite Jews who are slightly colored? This question becomes even more pressing when we realize that they are the only ones who are able to pronounce Hebrew in the most authentic way. Morag (2001, 31) mentions that the Yemenite tradition shows features of both the Tiberian and the Babylonian tradition. There appears to be no connection between the pre-Islamic Yemenite languages and the current Yemenite-Jewish pronunciation. In the Yemenite tradition, the close Hebrew (Yemenite) pronunciation of the two Hebrew vowels, חולם (*holam*; transliterated as *o*) and צירי (*tsere*; transliterated as *e* as in bed), was the Judean pronunciation as attested by biblical texts (personal communication by Yosef Tobi, of the University of Haifa). The way Ashkenazis pronounce Hebrew has little to do with the original pronunciation of Hebrew. An interesting observation actually, because the original pronunciation should have been passed on via the Hebrew prayers from father to son.

Interestingly, Yemenite Jews have little in common with Ashkenazic Jews genetically, as was first shown by Zoossmann-Diskin in 1997. Among Yemenite Jews, we find the African mtDNA lineages L1–L3a, but their frequency is rather low compared to those of non-Jews from the same region (Richards et al. 2003). The African lineages may have entered the Yemenite Jewish community during that period or maybe earlier as a result of commercial ties with sub-Saharan African countries. The presence of "non-Jewish" mtDNA haplotypes is normal though, as we have seen before.

Campbell et al. (2012) showed via primary component analysis (PCA) that Yemenite Jews did not form part of the Jewish cluster. They were distinct and statistically different as well. They write: "Like the Ethiopian Jews, this population was founded >2,000 yrs ago and was thought to be comprised mostly of local proselytes, which is reflected in the distinctive clustering of the population away from other Jewish groups and the mostly Middle Eastern ancestry present in this group." According to archaeological evidence, Jews lived in Yemen from the third century CE (Morag 2001, 22). The view that modern Yemenite Jews would be descendants of Himyarites is not correct, as I mentioned earlier (p. 52). It is likely that Campbell et al. are not familiar with the abovementioned features of Yemenite Jewry. Therefore, the idea that Yemenite Jews may be descendants of the Judeans, exactly because of these differences, may not have occurred to them.

The possibility that Yemenite Jews are straight descendants of Judeans or Israelites may be summarized by the combination of the following five points:

a. they have the most authentic pronunciation of Hebrew,
b. they are genetically different from the other groups of Jews (Zoossmann-Diskin 1997; Richards 2003),
c. they lived relatively isolated from the non-Jewish Yemenites,
d. their synagogal music is different from that of other groups of Jews (see van Straten 2011b, x–xii), and
e. among the Yemenite Jews, as among Greek, Indian, Armenian, and Samaritan communities that date back to antiquity, the same motifs in the chanting way of reciting are found (Morag 2001, 20–25).

During the fifties of the twentieth century, Yemenite Jews were discriminated against in Israel. This culminated in the kidnapping of newly born babies and putting them in Ashkenazic homes. The mother of the baby was told that the baby was very ill and that she should go home in the meantime. She was later informed that the baby had died. This practice came to light because Yemenite Jews don't look like Ashkenazis. Should this practice be mentioned in a scientific discussion? I think it should because it touches the essence of the origin of Ashkenazic Jewry, and it also shows to what kind of excessive behavior ideas about origin may lead. If a group of Jews with the above-mentioned qualities, who are not as white as Ashkenazis, and who are not genetically close to European Jews, would qualify best as being descendants of Judeans, what does this mean for the origin of Ashkenazic Jewry? By putting Yemenite babies in Ashkenazic homes, it would look as if Ashkenazis could also have these slightly colored babies. In schools, Yemenite children were discouraged to pronounce Hebrew the Yemenite way and use a pronunciation that is a mixture of the Oriental and Ashkenazic pronunciation. Ashkenazic rulers were clearly intent on removing the authentic way of pronouncing Hebrew to diminish their uneasy feelings about the Yemenite Jews.

A contemporary case of discrimination is that of Ethiopian Jews; again, Jews who are not white. In this case, it is a mix of religious and non-religious discrimination. On December 9, 2019, a lecture was delivered in the Orthodox Union Jerusalem World Center with the title: Falashas – Are They Jews? Falashas is a derogatory name for Ethiopian Jews. The answer of 9 rabbis was presented, 8 originally from Eastern Europe (Poland 2, Lithuania 3, Belarus 1, Russia 1, and Eastern Europe 1), and 1 Oriental, originally from Baghdad. The answer of the Ashkenazic rabbis was negative. Only the Oriental rabbi considered Ethiopian Jews as Jews. The chances that ultra-orthodox Jews would marry Ethiopian Jews are virtually non-existent, but the treatment of Ethiopian Jews by these kinds of rabbis leads to unnecessary harassment, as shown by a movie in which an Ashkenazic rabbi, checks whether or not an Ethiopian lady who works in a kosher catering company is Jewish. On the spot, the lady had to show papers that proved that she was Jewish. The lady did not carry her papers with her, got all upset, and started to cry. I wonder what would have happened if the lady had been white and English-speaking. Would she have been treated the same way? It is shameful that again Ashkenazis are involved in this kind of discriminatory behavior. I am not aware of the fact that ultra-orthodox rabbis have a monopoly on deciding who should be considered a Jew. Despite the fact that Israel's chief rabbinate recognized the Ethiopian Jewish community, this kind of harassment still takes place.

Another disturbing development, also occurring at present, is that today's rabbis want to use mtDNA, for example, K1a1b1a, to determine if someone who claims to be an Ashkenazic Jew is really a Jew. What we see here is that these rabbis are only interested in Jews belonging to their own DNA lineage, because then they qualify as being (Ashkenazic) Jewish. This development is clearly in disagreement with the original ruling that a convert is Jewish as well. The following is a good example. Around 1750, the Swedish family Granbom moved to Amsterdam and converted to Judaism. In 1797, one of their sons became rabbi of the orthodox-Jewish community *Adath Yeshurun*. According to his mtDNA (or his Y-chromosomal DNA), he would never have qualified as a Jew. This would hold for all Ashkenazis who are descendants of people who converted at some time in the past. This shows the absurdity of the new ruling. It also shows that converts who are (Ashkenazic) Jewish כדת וכדין (*ke-dath u-ke-din* – according to religion and Jewish law) all of a sudden are not Jewish anymore. Will they become second rate citizens? The rabbis who are in favor of this ruling do not seem to realize that religion does not depend on a lineage. Not only that, lineages like K1a1b1a are European lineages.

The DNA test is specifically meant for Russian immigrants. Let us assume the following: a Russian immigrant has a "non-kosher" mtDNA lineage because his/her maternal great-grandmother converted to Judaism. The immigrant would not pass the test, while the person is Ashkenazic Jewish according to rabbinical law. One may even compare the immigrant's situation with that of these same East European rabbis who deny the emigrant his Jewishness, with the only difference that the maternal foremother of the latter may have converted to Judaism much longer ago. This whole DNA test procedure is a terribly discriminating and also wrong procedure for testing Jewishness. Rabbis who decide who is Jewish should carefully read the article, mainly based on the Bible and Talmud, by Moshe Samet (1993, 316–343), who shows how easy it was to adopt the Jewish religion, shortly after the beginning of the Common Era. No test was necessary, it was enough that someone denied the idols (see also van Straten 2011, 142).

It is clear that research pertaining to the origin of today's Jews should become an objective activity again. This might not only have a positive influence on genetic research but on genealogical research as well.

The development of commercial firms that determine one's genealogical background via one's haplotype(s) sounds like a nice development. However, when one looks at some of the results, it is not clear whether some of these firms are not fraudulent. A good example is the family tree of a Levite composed by company X that goes back to famous rabbis (this the Levite probably found out himself), from there to King David, and ultimately to arch-father Abraham. Are the makers of such a family tree ignorant of Jewish history before the beginning of the Common Era, or do they just try to please people and make money this way? Maybe all Jews who are interested in their genetic history should first read *The Bible Unearthed* by Finkelstein and Silberman. This should give them enough insight to put firms that will take you to arch-father Abraham out of business.

In summary: sadly enough, the origin of East European Ashkenazis has become a political issue. The decision of someone being (Ashkenazic) Jewish has been made dependent on a genetic test, which is a violation of the original rabbinical ruling that one can become a Jew via conversion, and thus carry a completely different lineage from that (of the majority) of Ashkenazis.

I hope that the book has been of help to give the reader a better understanding of the early development of Ashkenazic Jewry. Moreover, I hope that, in addition, the epilogue has given some insights into the somewhat less scientific problems related to the origin of modern Jews in general and Ashkenazis specifically.

Bibliography

Adams, S.M., E. Bosch, P.L. Balaresque, et al. "The Genetic Legacy of Religious Diversity and Intolerance: Paternal Lineages of Christians, Jews, and Muslims in the Iberian Peninsula," *American Journal of Human Genetics* 83 (2008): 725–736.

Altbauer, M., and M. Taube. *The Five Biblical Scrolls in a Sixteenth-century Jewish Translation into Belorussian* (Vilnius Codex 262). Jerusalem: Israel Academy of Sciences and Humanities, 1992.

Ankori, Z. "Origins and History of Ashkenazi Jewry (8th to 18th Century)." In *Genetic Diseases among Ashkenazi Jews*, edited by R. M. Goodman and A. G. Motulsky, 49–46. New York: Raven Press, 1979.

Aptroot, M. "Yiddish Language and Ashkenazic Jews: a Perspective from Culture, Language, and Literature." *Genome Biology and Evolution* 8 (2016): 1948–1949.

Aslanov, C. "Hitgabshut shel ha-yidish ha-mizrahit" [The crystallization of Eastern Yiddish; text in Hebrew]. In *Toldot yehudey Rusia* [The History of the Russian Jews], edited by I. Bartal, 309–321. Jerusalem: Merkaz Zalman Shazar le-toldot Yísrael, 2010.

Atzmon, G., L. Hao, I. Pe'er, et al. "Abraham's Children in the Genome Era: Major Jewish Diaspora Populations Comprise Distinct Genetic Clusters with Shared Middle Eastern Ancestry." *American Journal of Human Genetics* 86 (2010): 850–859.

Avraham, A. 2010, http://www.yivoencyclopedia.org/article.aspx/Sephardim.

Bahlow, H. *Schlesisches Namenbuch*, Kitzingen/Main: Holzner Verlag, 1953.

Balanovsky, O., Kh. Dibirova, A. Dybo, et al. "Parallel Evolution of Genes and Languages in the Caucasus Region." *Molecular Biology and Evolution* 28 (2011): 2905–2920.

Baltrusch, E. "Die konstantinische *lex generalis* von 321 an die Stadt Köln und die Juden." In *Ein gefüllter Willkomm: Festschrift für Knut Schultz zum 65. Geburtstag*, edited by F. J. Felten, S. Irrgang, and K. Wesoly, 1–15. Aachen: Shaker, 2002.

Baron, S.W. *A Social and Religious History of the Jews.* New York: Columbia University Press, 1957–1976.

Bartal, I. "The Establishment of East European Jewry," In The Cambridge History of Judaism. Vol. 7: *The Early Modern World, 1500–1815*, edited by J. Karp and A. Sutcliffe, 226–256. Cambridge: Cambridge University Press, 2017.

Behar, D.M., D. Garrigan, M. E. Kaplan, et al. "Contrasting Patterns of Y Chromosome Variation in Ashkenazi Jewish and Host non-Jewish European Populations." *Human Genetics* 114 (2004a): 354–365.

Behar, D.M., M.F. Hammer, D. Garrigan et al. "MtDNA Evidence for a Genetic Bottleneck in the Early History of the Ashkenazi Jewish Population." *European Journal of Human Genetics* 12 (2004b):3 55–364.

Behar, D.M., E. Metspalu, T. Kivisild, et al. "The Matrilineal Ancestry of Ashkenazi Jewry: Portrait of a Recent Founder Event." *American Journal of Human Genetics* 78 (2006): 487–497.

Behar, D.M., E. Metspalu, T. Kivisild, et al. "Counting the Founders: The Matrilineal Genetic Ancestry of the Jewish Diaspora." *PloS One* 3 (2008): e2062.

Behar, D.M., M. Metspalu, Y. Baran, et al. "No Evidence from Genome-Wide Data of a Khazar Origin for the Ashkenazi Jews." *Human Biology Open Access Pre-Prints.* Paper 41. 2013.

Behar, D.M., L. Saag, M. Karmin, et al. "The Genetic Variation in the R1a Clade Among the Ashkenazi Levites' Y Chromosome." *Scientific Reports* 7 (2017): 14969.

https://doi.org/10.1515/9783110701388-012

Behar, D.M., M.G. Thomas, K. Skorecki, et al. “Multiple Origins of Ashkenazi Levites: Y Chromosome Evidence for Both Near Eastern and European Ancestries.” *American Journal of Human Genetics* 73 (2003): 768–779.

Behar, D.M., B. Yunusbayev, M. Metspalu, et al. “The Genome-wide Structure of the Jewish People.” *Nature* 466 (2010): 238–242.

Ben-Sasson, H.H. *A History of the Jewish People.* Cambridge: Harvard University Press, 1976.

Binstock, B., and S.A. Novoselsky. *Materialy o Estestvennom Dvizhenii Evreiskogo Naseleniya Evropeiskoi Rossii*, [Materials on the natural movement of the Jewish Population of European Russia; text in Russian]. Petrograd, 1915.

Botticini, M., Z. Eckstein and A. Vaturi. “The Chosen Many: Population Growth and Jewish Childcare in Central-Eastern Europe, 1500–1930.” Discussion Paper No.4–16, The Pinhas Sapir Center for Development, Tel Aviv University, 2016.

Boulnois, L. *The silk road.* London: George Allen & Unwin, 1966.

Bowman, S.B. *The Jews of Byzantium, 1204–1453*, University, AB: University of Alabama Press, 1985.

Bradman, N., M. Thomas and D. Goldstein. “The Genetic Origins of Old Testament Priests.” In *America Past, America Present: Genes and Languages in the Americas and Beyond*, edited by C. Renfrew, 31–44. Cambridge, UK: The McDonald Institute for Archaeological Research, 2000.

Breuer, M., and M. Graetz. *Deutsch-jüdische Geschichte in der Neuzeit.* Vol. 1: *Tradition und Aufklärung 1600–1780.* Munich: Beck, 1996.

Bürstenbinder, J. *Judenschutz und Eigennutz; Auseinandersetzungen um die Juden an der Ostgrenze des Römisch-Deutschen Reiches im 13. und 14. Jahrhundert.* Berlin: Südwestdeutscher Verlag für Hochschulschriften, 2010.

Campbell, C.L. “North African Jewish and Non-Jewish Populations Form Distinctive, Orthogonal Clusters.” *Proceedings of the National Academy of Sciences* 109 (2012): 13865–13870.

Carmi, S., K.Y. Hui, E. Kochav, et al. “Sequencing an Ashkenazi Reference Panel Supports Population-targeted Personal Genomics and Illuminates Jewish and European Origins.” *Nature Commununications* 5 (2014): 4835.

Caro, G. *Sozial- und Wirtschaftsgeschichte der Juden im Mittelalter und der Neuzeit.* Vol. 1: *Das frühere und das hohe Mittelalter.* Leipzig: Fock, 1920.

Cavalli-Sforza, L.L., and D. Carmelli. “The Ashkenazi Gene Pool: Interpretations.” In *Genetic diseases in Ashkenazi Jews*, edited by R. M. Goodman and A. G. Motulsky, 93–104. New York: Raven Press, 1979.

Chiaroni, J., R.J. King, N.M. Myres, et al. “The Emergence of Y-chromosome Haplotype J1e Among Arabic-speaking Populations.” *European Journal of Human Genetics* 18 (2010): 348–353.

Cinnioglu, C., R. King, T. Kivisild, et al. “Excavating Y-chromosome Haplotype Strata in Anatolia.” *Human Genetics* 114 (2004): 127–148.

Coale, A.J., and P. Demeny. *Regional Model Life Tables and Stable Population.* Princeton: Princeton University Press, 1966.

Cohen, S.J.D. *The Beginnings of Jewishness: Boundaries, Varieties, Uncertainties.* Berkeley: University of California Press, 1999.

Costa M.D., J.P. Pereira, M. Pala, et al. "A Substantial Prehistoric European Ancestry amongst Ashkenazi Maternal Lineages." *Nature Communications* 4 (2013): 2543. doi: 10.1038/ncomms3543.
Dan'shin, D.I. "The Jewish Community of Phanagoria," *Ancient Civilizations* 3 (1966): 133–150.
Das, R., P. Wexler, M. Piroozna, and E. Elhaik. "Localizing Ashkenazic Jews in Primeval Villages in the Ancient Iranian Lands of Ashkenaz." *Genome Biology and Evolution* 8 (2016): 1132–1149.
DellaPergola, S. "Alcuni aspetti quantitative della distribuzione del cognomen fra gli ebrei in Italia." *Annunario di Studi Ebraici* 10 (1984): 65–86.
DellaPergola, S. "Some Fundamentals of Jewish Demographic History." iIn *Papers in Jewish Demography 1997*, edited by S. DellaPergola and J. Even, 11–33. Jerusalem: Avraham Harman Institute of Contemporary Jewry, 2001.
Department of Justice, Immigration and Naturalization Service. (2007). http://www.infoplease.com/ipa/A0201398.html. Immigrants to U.S. by country of origin.
Dietz, A. *Stammbuch der Frankfurter Juden: geschichtliche Mitteilungen über die Frankfurter jüdischen Familien von 1349–1849 nebst eine Plane der Judengasse.* Frankfurt am Main, 1907.
Dittmann, R. "West Slavic Canaanite Glosses in Medieval Hebrew Manuscripts." *Judaica. Beiträge zum Verstehen des Judentums* 73, no. 2–3 (2017): 234–283.
Dopsch, A. *Wirtschafliche und soziale Grundlagen der europäischen Kulturentwicklung aus der Zeit von Cäsar bis auf Karl den Grossen.* Vol. 1. Vienna: Seidel, 1923.
Eggers, E. *Sprachwandel und Sprachmischung im Jiddischen.* Frankfurt am Main: Lang, 1988.
Ehret, Chr. "Language Change and the Material Correlates of Language and Ethnic Shift." *Antiquity* 62 (1988): 564–573.
Elhaik, E. "The Missing Link of Jewish European Ancestry: Contrasting the Rhineland and the Khazarian Hypothesis." *Genome Biology and Evolution* 5 (2012): 61–74.
Encyclopaedia Judaica. Vol. 6, Ephesos. Berlin: Verlag Eschkol, 1930.
Encyclopedia Judaica. Vol. 5. Detroit: Thomson Gale, 2007.
Encyclopedia of Jews in the Islamic World. Vol. 3. Ottoman Empire. Leiden/Boston, 2010.
Engelman, U. Z. "Sources of Jewish Statistics." In *The Jews: their History , Culture, and Religion.* Vol. 2, 3rd ed., edited by L. Finkelstein, 1510–1535. New York, 1960.
Epstein, M.A. *The Ottoman Jewish Communities and their Role in the Fifteenth and Sixteenth Centuries*, Freiburg: Schwarz, 1980.
Faber, A., and R.D. King. "Yiddish and the Settlement History of Ashkenazic Jews." *The Mankind Quarterly* 24 (1984): 393–425.
Falk, R. *Zionism and the Biology of the Jews*, e-book. 2017.
Farley R., and J. Haaga. *1607–1820: The American people: census 2000.* New York, 2005.
Feder, J., O. Ovadia, B. Glaser, and D. Mishmar. "Ashkenazi Jewish mtDNA Haplogroup Distribution Varies Among Distinct Subpopulations: Lessons of Population Substructure in a Closed Group." *European Journal of Human Genetics* 15 (2007): 498–500.
Feist, S. "Sind die Juden eine Rasse?" *Zeitschrift für Demographie und Statistik der Juden*, new series 4 (1927): 6–11.
Fernández, E., A. Pérez-Pérez, C. Gamba, et al. "Ancient DNA Analysis of 8000 B.C. Near Eastern Farmers Supports an Early Neolithic Pioneer Maritime Colonization of Mainland

Europe through Cyprus and the Aegean Islands." *PloS Genetics* 10, no. 6 (2014): e1004401.
Finkelstein, I. "Ethnicity and Origin of the Iron I Settlers in the Highlands of Canaan: Can the Real Israel Stand Up?" *Biblical Archaeologist* 59, no. 4 (1996): 198–212.
Finkelstein, I. *The Forgotten Kingdom; the Archaeology and History of Northern Israel.* Atlanta: Society of Biblical Literature, 2013.
Finkelstein, I. and N.A. Silberman. *The Bible Unearthed: Archaeology's New Vision of Ancient Israel and the Origin of its Sacred Texts.* New York: Touchstone, 2002.
Finkelstein, I. and N.A. Silberman. *David and Solomon.* New York: Free Press, 2006.
Finocchio, A. "A Finely Resolved Phylogeny of Y Chromosome HgJ Illuminates the Processes of Phoenician and Greek Colonizations in the Mediterranean." *Scientific Reports* 8 (2018): 7465.
Fishberg, M. "Zur Frage der Herkunft des blonden Elements im Judentum." *Zeitschrift für Demographie und Statistik der Juden* 3 (1907): 25–30.
Fishberg, M. *The Jews: a Study of Race and Environment.* London: Walter Scott, 1911.
Flegontov, P., A. Kassian, M.G. Thomas, et al. "Pitfalls of the Geographic Population Structure (GPS) Approach Applied to Human Genetic History: a Case Study of Ashkenazi Jews." *Genome Biology and Evolution* 8 (2016): 2259–2265.
Fremersdorf, F. "Jahresbericht des staatlichen Vertrauensmannes für kulturgeschichtliche Bodenaltertümer im Stadtkreis Köln vom 1. April 1937 bis 31. März 1938." *Bonner Jahrbuch* 143/144 (1938/39): 453–455.
Frishman, A. *Ha-ashkenazim ha-r'ishonim* [the first Ashkenazis; text in Hebrew]. Tel Aviv: ha-kibuts ha-me-uhad, 2008.
Gechter, M., and S. Schütte. "Ursprung und Voraussetzungen des mittelalterlichen Rathauses und seiner Umgebung." In *Köln: Das gotische Rathaus und seine historische Umgebung,* edited by W. Geis and U. Krings, 69–195. Cologne: J.P. Bachem Verlag, 2000.
Gladstein, A.L., and M.F. Hammer. "Substructured Population Growth in the Ashkenazi Jews Inferred with Approximate Bayesian Computation." *Molecular Biology and Evolution* 36 (2019): 1162–1171.
Goeje, M.J. de. *Kitâb al-masâlik wa'l-mamâlik* (Liber viarum et regnorum). Leiden: Brill, 1889.
Guha, S., J.A. Rosenfeld, A.K. Malhotra, et al. "Implications for Health and Disease in the Genetic Signature of the Ashkenazi Jewish Population." *Genome Biology* 13 (2012): r2.
Haak, W., I. Lazaridis, N. Patterson, et al. "Massive Migration from the Steppe Was a Source for Indo-European Languages in Europe." *Nature* 522 (2015): 207–211.
Haber, M., C. Doumet-Serhal, Ch. Scheib, et al. "Continuity and Admixture in the last Five Millennia of Levatine History from Ancient Canaanite and Present-day Lebanese Genome Sequences." *American Journal of Human Genetics* 101 (2017): 1–9.
Halpern, I. "The Jews in Eastern Europe." In *The Jews: their History, Culture and Religion.* Vol. 1, 3rd ed., edited by L. Finkelstein, 287–320. New York: Harper, 1960.
Hammer, M.F., A.J. Redd, E.T. Wood, et al. "Jewish and Middle Eastern Non-Jewish Populations Share a Common Pool of Y-Chromosome Biallelic Haplotypes." *Proceedings of the National Academy of Sciences USA* 97 (2000): 6769–6774.
Hammer, M.F., D.M. Behar, T.M. Karafet, et al. "Extended Y Chromosome Haplotypes Resolve Multiple and Unique Lineages of the Jewish Priesthood." *Human Genetics* 126 (2009): 707–717.

Harck, O. *Archäologische Studien zum Judentum in der europäischen Antike und dem zentraleuropäischen Mittelalter.* Petersberg: Michael Imhof Verlag, 2014.
Harkavy, A.E. *Ha-yehudim u-sfat ha-slavim* [The Jews and the language of the Slavs; text in Hebrew]. Vilnius: Romm, 1867.
Heyd, U. "The Jewish Communities of Istanbul in the Seventeenth Century." *Oriens* 6 (1953): 299 – 314.
Hopkirk, P. *Foreign Devils on the Silk Road.* London: John Murray, 1980.
Horowitz, A. *Sefer yesh nohalin* [there are heirs; text in Hebrew]. Amsterdam: Athias, 1701.
Horowitz, H. "Die Familie Horowitz in Prag im 16. Jahthundert." *Zeitschrift für die Geschichte der Juden in der Tschechoslowakei* 2 (1931): 89 – 105.
Hundert, G.D. "Poland: Paradisus Judaeorum." *Journal of Jewish Social Studies* 48 (1997): 335 – 348.
Inalcik, H. "The Ottoman Economic Mind and Aspects of the Ottoman Economy." In *Studies in the Economic History of the Middle East*, edited by M.A. Cook, 207–218. London: Oxford University Press, 1970.
Jeffery, L.H. *Archaic Greece the City-States c. 700 – 500 B.C.* London: Ernest Benn, 1976.
JewishEncyclopedia.com. Ravenna.
Jewishhistory.org.il. 846.
Jewish Surnames of Turkey. http://www.angelfire.com/wy/yaw/jewish.htm.
Kabuzan, V.M. *Narody Rossii v pervoi polovine XIX v.: Chislennost I etnicheskij sostav*, [Peoples of Russia in the first half of the XIX century: population and ethnic composition; text in Russian]. Moscow, 1992.
Karniel, J. *Die Toleranzpolitik Kaiser Josephs II.* Gerlingen: Bleicher, 1986.
Katz, D. "Hebrew, Aramaic and the Rise of Yiddish." In *Readings in the Sociology of the Jewish Languages*, edited by J.A. Fishman, 85 – 103. Leiden: Brill, 1985.
King, R.D. "Migration and Linguistics as Illustrated by Yiddish." In *Reconstructing Languages and Cultures*, edited by E. C. Polomé and W. Winter, 419 – 439. Berlin/New York: Mouton de Gruyter, 1992.
Knipper, C., A. Mittnik, K. Massy, et al. "Female Exogamy and Gene Pool Diversification at the Transition from the Final Neolithic to the Early Bronze Age in Central Europe." *Proceedings of the National Academy of Sciences* 144 (2017): 10083 – 10088.
Kober, A. "Cöln." In *Germania Judaica* [I]; *Von den ältesten Zeiten bis 1238*, edited by I. Elbogen, A. Freimann and H. Tykocinski, 69–85. Breslau: Verlag M & H Marcus, 1934.
Kober, A. "Otto Kraus: Feststellungen bei den Ausgrabungsarbeiten auf dem Gelände des alten israelitischen Friedhofe am Bahnhof vor den Bonner Tor, Cologne, 1922 (manuscript)." *American Academy for Jewish Research, Proceedings* 15 (1945): 3 – 14, 81 – 83.
Kochelenko, G., and V. Kouznetsov. "La Colonization Grecque du Bosphore Cimmérien." In *Le Pont-Euxin vu par les Grecs: sources écrites et archeology*, symposium de Vani (Colchide), septembre-octobre, edited by T. Khartchilava and E. Geny, 8 – 82. Besaçon: Université de Franche-Comté, 1987.
Koestler, A. *The Thirteenth Tribe.* New York: Random House, 1976.
Kopelman, N.M., L. Stone, Ch. Wang, et al. "Genomic Microsatellites Identify Shared Jewish Ancestry Intermediate Between Middle Eastern and European Populations." *BMC Genet*ics 10 (2009): 80.

Kosmin, B. A. and S. Waterman. "The Use and Misuse of Distinctive Jewish names." In *Papers in Jewish Demography 1985*, edited by U. O. Schmelz and S. DellaPergola, 1–10. Jerusalem: Association for Jewish Demography and Statistics, 1989.

Kraabel, A.T. "The Diaspora Synagogue: Archaeological Epigraphic Evidence since Sukenik." In *Ancient synagogues; historical analysis and archaeological discovery*, edited by D. Urman and P.V.M. Flesher, 95–126. Second impression. Leiden: Brill, 1995.

Kutschera, H. Freiherr von. *Die Chasaren*. Vienna: Holzhausen, 1910.

Landau, M. Review of *Khazaria: toldot mamlakhah yehudit be-eyropah* [Khazaria: History of a Jewish Kingdom in Europe; text in Hebrew], by N. Polak. *Kiriat sefer* 21 (1944): 19–24.

Lestschinsky, J. "Jewish Migrations, 1840–1956." In *The Jews: their History, Culture, and Religion*. Vol. 2, 3rd ed., edited by L. Finkelstein, 1536–1596. New York, 1960.

Leuchter, M. *The Levites and the Boundaries of Israelite Identity*. New York: Oxford University Press, 2017.

Levinskaya, I.A. *The Book of Acts in its Diaspora Setting*. Grand Rapids: William B Eerdmans Publishing Co., 1996.

Levinskaya, I.A. and S.R. Tokhtas'yev, "Jews and Jewish Names in the Bosporan Kingdom." In *Studies on the Jewish Diaspora in the Hellenistic and Roman Periods*, edited by B. Isaac and A. Oppenheimer, 55–73. Tel Aviv: Ramot Publishing, 1996.

Levy, A. *The Jews of the Ottoman Empire*. Princeton, N. J.: Darwin Press, 1994

Lewis, B. *The Jews of Islam*. Princeton, N.J.: Princeton University Press, 1987

Lewis, D.M. *Selected Papers in Greek and Near Eastern History*. Cambridge: Cambridge University Press, 1997.

Liverani, M. *Israel's History and the History of Israel*. London: Equinox Publishing Ltd, 2005.

Livi-Bacci, M. *The Population of Europe: A History*. Translated by Cynthia de Nardi Ipsen and Carl Ipsen. Oxford: Blackwell, 1999.

Maddison, A. *The World Economy a Millennial Perspective*. Paris: Development Centre of the Organisation for Economic Co-operation and Development, 2001.

Marmorstein, A. 2016, "Does the Horowitz Family from Bohemia Really Descend from the Benvenisti Halevy Family from Spain? [AB-067]." https://avotaynuonline.com/2016/03/does-the-horowitz-family-from-bohemia-really-descend-from-the-benvenisti-halevy-family-from-spain/.

McEvedy, C., and R. Jones. *Atlas of World Population History*. London: Allen Lane, 1978.

Menache, S. "Tartars, Jews, Saracens and the Jewish-Mongol 'Plot' of 1241." *History. A Quarterly Magazine and Review for the Teacher, the Student, and the Expert* 81 (1996): 319–342.

Mieses, M. *Die Jiddische Sprache*. Berlin/Vienna: Verlag Benjamin Harz, 1924.

Morag, Sh. *Masoroth ha-lashon ha-'ivrith ve-ha-lashon ha-'aramith she-be-pi yehudei theman* [Traditions of the Hebrew language and the Aramaic language according to the Jews of Yemen], edited by Y. Tobi. Tel Aviv: Afikim, 2001.

Motulsky, A.G. "Jewish Diseases and Origins." *Nature Genetics* 9 (1995): 99–101.

Müller, G., and Th. Frings. *Germania Romana II: Dreissig Jahre Forschung romanische Wörter*. Halle (Saale): Niemeyer, 1968.

Na'aman, N. "Yeno'am." *Tel Aviv* 4 (1977): 168–177.

Nebel, A., D. Filon, M. Faerman, et al. "Y Chromosome Evidence for a Founder Effect in Ashkenazi Jews." *European Journal of Human Genetics* 13 (2005): 388–391.

Need, A.C., D. Kasperavičiūtė, E.T. Cirulli, and D.B. Goldstein. "A Genome-wide Genetic Signature of Jewish Ancestry Perfectly Separates Individuals with and without Full Jewish Ancestry in a Large Random Sample of European Americans." *Genome Biology* 10 (2009): R7.

Nogueiro, I., J. Teixeira, A. Amorim, et al. "Echoes from Sepharad: Signatures on the Maternal Gene Pool of Crypto-Jewish Descendants." *European Journal of Human Genetics* (2014): 1–7.

Olalde, I., S. Mallick, N. Patterson, et al. "The Genomic History of the Iberian Peninsula over the Past 8000 Years." *Science* 363 (2019): 1230–1234.

Ostrer, H. *Legacy: a Genetic History of the Jewish People.* Oxford: Oxford University Press, 2012.

Ostrer, H., and K. Skorecki. "The Population Genetics of the Jewish People." *Human Genetics* 132 (2013): 119–127.

Palamara, P.F., T. Lencz, A. Darvasi, and I. Pe'er. "Length Distributions of Identity by Descent Reveal Fine-Scale Demographic History." *American Journal of Human Genetics* 91 (2012): 809–822.

Passarino, G., O. Semino, Ch. Magri, et al. "The 49a,f Haplotype 11 is a New Marker of the Eu19 Lineage that Traces Migrations from Northern Regions of the Black Sea." *Human Immunology* 62 (2001): 922–932.

Philo J.A. *Legatio ad Caium.* Paris: Éditions du Cerf, 1972.

Polak, A.N. "Hitgayrut ha-kuzarim" [The conversion of the Khazars; text in Hebrew]. *Tsion* 6 (1941): 106–112.

Rhodes, P.J. *A History of the Classical Greek World: 478–323 BC.* Malden, MA: Blackwell, 2006.

Reinach, S. "Inscription grecque de Smyrne." *Revue des Études Juives* 7 (1883): 161–166.

Richards, M.B., Ch. Rengo, F. Cruciani, et al. "Extensive Female-Mediated Gene Flow from Sub-Saharan Africa into Near Eastern and Arab Populations." *American Journal of Human Genetics* 72 (2003):1058–1064.

Risch, N. "Molecular Epidemiology of Tay-Sachs Disease." *Advances in Genetics* 44 (2001): 233–252.

Rodrigues Pereira, H., and H. Snel. "Joodse huwelijken in Amsterdam." *Misjpoge* 32 (2019): 2–13.

Rootsi, S., D.M. Behar, M. Järve, et al. "Phylogenetic Applications of Whole Y-chromosome Sequences and the Near Eastern Origin of Ashkenazi Levites." *Nature Communications* 4 (2013): 2928.

Rootsi, S., N.M. Myres, A.A. Lin, et al. "Distinguishing the Co-ancestries of Haplogroup G Y-chromosomes in the Populations of Europe and the Caucasus." *European Journal of Human Genetics* 20 (2012): 1275–1282.

Rotner, D.N. "He'arot le-shoshelet mishpahat Horwits – ha-leviim [The Dynasty of the Horowits family – the Levites; text in Hebrew]." *Kovets "Bet Aharon ve-Yisrael* 113 (2004): 155–161.

Rozanes, S.A. *Divre yeme Yisrael be-Togarma: 'al pi meqorim yesharim* [The History of the Jews in Turkey; text in Hebrew]. Vol. 1. Husiyatin: F. Qawaleg, 1908.

Rupin, A. *Sociologie der Juden*, Vol. 1: *Die sociale Struktur der Juden.* Berlin: Jüdischer Verlag, 1930.

Rutgers, L.V. "Reflections on the Demography of the Jewish Community of Ancient Rome." In *Les cités de l'Italie tardo-antique (IVe-VIe siècle)*, edited by M. Ghilardi and Chr. J. Goddard, 1–14. Rome: École Française de Rome, 2006.

Samet, M. "Ha-giur be-me'ot ha-r'ishonot la-sfirah" [Conversions to Judaism during the first centuries C.E.; text in Hebrew]. In *Yehudim ve-yahadut bi-mey bayit sheni, ha-mishnah ve-ha-talmud.* Jerusalem, 1993.

Sand, Sh. *The Invention of the Jewish People.* London/New York: Verso, 2009.

Santachiara Benerecetti, A.S., O. Semino, G. Passarino, et al. "The Common, Near-Eastern Origin of Ashkenazi and Sephardi Jews Supported by Y-chromosome Similarity." *Annals of Human Genetics* 57 (1993): 55–64.

Sassoon, D.S. *A history of the Jews in Baghdad.* Letchworth: S.D. Sassoon, 1949.

Schuler, A. *Der römische Friedhof an der Sechtemer Strasse im Kölner Süden.* Kölner Jahrbuch 35, 2002 (ersch. 2004): 437–570.

Schütte, S. "Der Almemor der Kölner Synagoge um 1270/80: Gotische Klein-architektur aus der Kölner Dombauhütte." In Colonia Romanica Jahrbuch des Fördervereins Romanische Kirchen Köln e. V., vol. 13, 188–215. Cologne: Greven Verlag, 1998.

Schütte, S., and M. Gechter. *Von der Ausgrabung zum Museum – Kölner Archäologie zwischen Rathaus und Praetorium; Ergebnisse und Materialien 2006–2012.* Vienna: Stadt Köln, 2012.

Sergi, O. "Rethinking Israel and the Kingdom of Saul." In *Rethinking Israel: Studies in the History and Archaeology of Ancient Israel in Honor of Israel Finkelstein*, edited by O. Lipschits, Y. Gadot, and M.J. Adams, 371–388. Winona Lake, IN: Eisenbrauns, 2017.

Silber, M.K. "The Making of Habsburg Jewry in the Long Eighteenth Century." In *The Early Modern World, 1500–1815*, edited by J. Karp and A. Sutcliffe, 763–797. Cambridge: Cambridge University Press, 2017.

Silbergleit, H. *Die Bevölkerungs- und Berufsverhältnisse der Juden im deutsche Reich auf Grund von amtlichen Materialien. I: Freistaat Preussen.* Berlin, 1930.

Simon, G. 2006. https://homepages.uni-tuebingen.de/gerd.simon/VorgeschDossiers.pdf.

Simonsohn, Sh. *The Jews in Sicily*, vol 1, *383–1300*, Leiden: Brill, 1997.

Simonsohn, Sh. *The Jews of Italy: antiquity.* Leiden: Brill, 2014.

Skorecki, K., S. Selig, Sh. Blazer, et al. "Y Chromosomes of Jewish priests." *Nature* 385 (1997): 32.

Slatkin, M. "A population-genetic Test of Founder Effects and Implications for Ashkenazi Jewish Diseases." *American Journal of Human Genetics* 75 (2004): 282–293.

Stampfer, Sh. "Violence and Migration of Ashkenazi Jews to Eastern Europe." In *Jews in East European Borderlands: Essays in honor of John D. Klier*, edited by E.M. Avrutin and H. Murav, 127–146. Boston: Academic Studies Press, 2012.

Stampfer, Sh. "Did the Khazars Convert to Judaism?" *Jewish Social Studies* 19, no. 3 (2013): 1–72.

Starr, J. *The Byzantine Empire 641–1204.* Athens: Verlag der Byzantinisch-Neugriechischen Jahrbücher, 1939.

Stern, M. *Greek and Latin Authors on Jews and Judaism.* Jerusalem: Israel Academy of Sciences and Humanities, 1980.

Straten, J. van "Jewish Migrations from Germany to Poland: the Rhineland Hypothesis Revisited." *The Mankind Quarterly* 44 (2004): 367–383.

Straten, J. van "Early Modern Polish Jewry: The Rhineland Hypothesis Revisited." *Historical Methods* 40 (2007): 39–50.

Straten, J. van *De herkomst van de Asjkenazische joden: de controverse opgelost.* Bennekom: self-published, 2009.

Straten, J. van *The Origin of Ashkenazi Jewry: The Controversy Unraveled.* Berlin/New York: de Gruyter, 2011a.

Straten, J. van "The Yemenite Jews: an Exceptional Group?" In *Mittuv Yosef: Yosef Tobi Jubilee Volume*, vol. 2: *The Jews of Yemen: History and Culture*, edited by A. Oettinger and D. Bar-Maoz, ix–xvii. Haifa: University of Haifa, 2011b.

Straten, J. van "The Origin of East European Ashkenazim via a Southern Route." *Aschkenas* 27 (2017): 239–270.

Straten, J. van, and H. Snel. "The Jewish 'Demographic Miracle' in Nineteenth-Century Europe: Fact or Fiction?" *Historical Methods* 39 (2006): 123–131.

Tacitus, P.C. *Annalivm ab excessv divi Avgvsti libri*; recognovit brevique adnotatione critica instrvxit. Oxford: E typographeo Clarendoniano, 1906.

Talmon, S. "What's a Calendar? Calendar Conformity. Calendar Controversy, and Calendar Reform in Ancient and Medieval Judaism." In *Seeking out the wisdom of the ancients; essays offered to honor Michael V. Fox on the occasion of his sixty-fifth birthday*, edited by R. L. Troxel, K.G. Friebel, and D.R. Magary, 451–460. Winona Lake: Eisenbraun, 2005.

Ta-Shma, I.M. "Asher b. Yehiel." In *Medieval Jewish Civilization: An Encyclopedia*, edited by N. Roth. New York & London: Routledge, 2003.

Theophanes Abbas Agri et Confessor. *Theophanis Chronographia* [historical account of Thiophanes; text in Greek and Latin]. Bonn: Ed. Weber, 1839.

Thomas, M.G., K. Skorecki, H. Ben-Ami, et al. "Origins of Old Testament Priests." *Nature* 394 (1998):138–140.

Thomas, M.G., M.E. Weale, A.L. Jones, et al. "Founding Mothers of Jewish Communities: Geographically Separated Jewish Groups Were Independently Founded by Very Few Female Ancestors." *American Journal of Human Genetics* 70 (2002): 1411–1420.

Tian, J.-Y., H.-W. Wang, Y.-Ch Li, et al. "A Genetic Contribution from the Far East into Ashkenazi Jews via the Ancient Silk Road." *Scientific Reports* 5 (2015): 8377.

Toch, M. "Jewish Migrations to, within and from Medieval Germany." In *Le migrazioni in Europa, secc. Xiii–xviii: Atti della 'Venticinquesima Settimana di studi' 3–8 maggio 1993*, edited by S. Cavaciocchi, 639–652. Florence: Le Monnier, 1994.

Toch, M. *Die Juden im mittelalterlichen Reich.* Munich: Oldenbourg, 1998.

Toch, M. *Dunkle Jahrhunderte; Gab es ein jüdisches Frühmittelalter?* 3. "Arye Maimon-Vortrag" an der Universität Trier, November 15, 2000. 2001.

Toch, M. *The Economic History of European Jews. Late Antiquity and Early Middle Ages.* Leiden/Boston: Brill, 2013.

Toch, M. "The Emergence of the Medieval Jewish Diaspora(s) of Europe from the Ninth to the Twelfth Centuries, with Some Thoughts on Historical DNA Studies." In *Regional Identities and Cultures of Medieval Jews*, edited by J. Castano, T. Fishman, and E. Kanarfogel, 21–35. London, 2018.

Toury, J. *Soziale und politische Geschichte der Juden in Deutschland 1847–1871. Zwischen Revolution, Reaktion und Emanzipation.* Düsseldorf: Droste, 1977.

Trombetta, B., E. D'Atanasio, A. Massaia, et al. "Phylogeographic Refinement and Large Scale Genotyping of Human Y Chromosome Haplogroup E Provide New Insights into the

Dispersal of Early Pastoralists in the African Continent." *Genome Byology and Evolution* 7 (2015): 1940–1950.
Weinreich, M. *History of the Yiddish Language.* Chicago/London: University of Chicago Press, 1980.
Weinryb, B.D. *The Jews of Poland: A Social Economic History of the Jewish Community in Poland from 1100–1800.* Philadelphia: Jewish Publication Society of America, 1972/3.
Wexler, P. "Yiddish—The Fifteenth Slavic Language: A Study of Partial Language Shift from Jewish-Sorbian to German." *International Journal of the Sociology of Language* 91 (1991): 9–150.
Xue, J., T. Lencz, A. Darvasi, et al. "The Time and Place of European Admixture in Ashkenazi Jewish History." *PloS Genetics* 13, no. 4 (2017): e1006644.
Yacobi, D., and F.L. Bedford. "Evidence of Early Gene Flow Between Ashkenazi Jews and non-Jewish Europeans in mitochondrial DNA haplogroup H7." *Journal of Genetic Genealogy* 8 (2016): 21–34.
Zalloua, P.A., D.E. Platt, M. El Sibai, et al. "Identifying Genetic Traces of Historical Expansions: Phoenician Footprints in the Mediterranean." *American Journal of Human Genetics* 83 (2008): 633–642.
Zegura, S.L. "High Resolution SNPs and Microsatellite Haplotypes Point to a Single, Recent Entry of Native American Y Chromosomes into the Americas." *Molecular Biology and Evolution* 21 (2004): 164–175.
Zinberg, I. *A History of Jewish Literature*, Vol. 6: *The German-Polish Cultural Center.* Cincinnati: Hebrew Union College Press, 1975.
Zoossmann-Diskin, A. *Tracing the Roots and Unfolding the Ethno-Historical Relationships of Jewish Communities by Means of DNA and Protein Electrophoretic Markers.* PhD diss., Tel-Aviv University, Tel-Aviv, 1997.
Zoossmann-Diskin, A. "Are today's Jewish Priests Descended from the Old Ones?" *HOMO* 51 (2000): 156–162.
Zoossmann-Diskin, A. "The origin of Eastern European Jews Revealed by Autosomal, Sex Chromosomal and mtDNA Polymorphisms." *Biology Direct* 5 (2010): 57.
Zoossmann-Diskin, A. A. Joel, M. Liron, et al. "Protein Electrophoretic Markers in Israel: Compilation of Data and Genetic Affinities." *Annals of Human Biology* 29 (2002): 142–175.
Zuckerman, C. "On the Date of the Khazar's Conversion to Judaism and the Chronology of the Kings of the Rus' Oleg and Igor: a Study of the Anonymous Khazar Letter from the Genizah of Cairo." *Revue des Études Byzantines* 53 (1995): 237–270.
Zunz, L. *Die Ritus des synagogalen Gottesdienstes, geschichtlich entwickelt.* Berlin: J. Springer, 1859.

Index

https://doi.org/10.1515/9783110701388-013